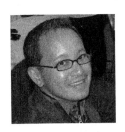

Don S. Di:  : University of F ry. He
trained in ospital
and in med ; Can-
cer Center MW01012728 Award
from the American Society of Clinical Oncology for work on
platinum drug resistance. He later joined the Developmental
Therapeutics faculty and Gynecology Disease Management Team of Memorial
Sloan-Kettering Cancer Center. In 2003 he left New York City and assumed his
current role as the director of medical oncology for the Program in Women's Oncology of Women & Infants' Hospital of Rhode Island. In 2005 he helped establish the state's first Center for Sexuality, Intimacy, and Fertility for women with
cancer. In 2005 he was elected Fellow of the American College of Physicians. He
also serves as medical director of the Program's Integrative Care Program. Nation-
ally, he continues to pursue research in the novel treatments of both breast and
gynecological cancers and is active in the Gynecologic Oncology Group, serving
on Phase I, Developmental Therapeutics, and Cervix committees. Currently he is
the president of the National Consortium of Breast Centers.

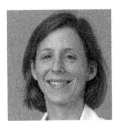

Linda R. Duska, MD, is an associate professor of obstetrics
and gynecology in the Division of Gynecologic Oncology at
the University of Virginia (UVA) where she is also the gynecologic oncology fellowship director. Dr. Duska received her
doctor of medicine from the New York University School of
Medicine and completed her residency in obstetrics and gynecology at the Johns Hopkins Hospital in Baltimore, MD.
Upon completion of her fellowship in gynecologic oncology at Massachusetts
General Hospital (MGH) in Boston, she joined the gynecologic oncology staff at
the Massachusetts General Hospital and was a member of the faculty of Harvard
University for 10 years prior to relocating to UVA.

100 Questions & Answers About Uterine Cancer

Don S. Dizon, MD, FACP

Director of Medical Oncology and Integrative Care
Co-Director, The Center for Sexuality, Intimacy and Fertility
Program in Women's Oncology
Women & Infants' Hospital
Assistant Professor
Department of Obstetrics & Gynecology and Medicine
The Warren Alpert Medical School of Brown University
Providence, RI

Linda R. Duska, MD

Associate Professor of Obstetrics and Gynecology
Fellowship Director
Gynecologic Oncology
University of Virginia
Charlottesville, VA

JONES AND BARTLETT PUBLISHERS
Sudbury, Massachusetts
BOSTON   TORONTO   LONDON   SINGAPORE

World Headquarters

Jones and Bartlett Publishers
40 Tall Pine Drive
Sudbury, MA 01776
978-443-5000
info@jbpub.com
www.jbpub.com

Jones and Bartlett Publishers
Canada
6339 Ormindale Way
Mississauga, Ontario L5V 1J2
Canada

Jones and Bartlett Publishers
International
Barb House, Barb Mews
London W6 7PA
United Kingdom

Jones and Bartlett's books and products are available through most bookstores and online booksellers. To contact Jones and Bartlett Publishers directly, call 800-832-0034, fax 978-443-8000, or visit our website, www.jbpub.com.

Substantial discounts on bulk quantities of Jones and Bartlett's publications are available to corporations, professional associations, and other qualified organizations. For details and specific discount information, contact the special sales department at Jones and Bartlett via the above contact information or send an email to specialsales@jbpub.com.

The authors, editor, and publisher have made every effort to provide accurate information. However, they are not responsible for errors, omissions, or for any outcomes related to the use of the contents of this book and take no responsibility for the use of the products and procedures described. Treatments and side effects described in this book may not be applicable to all people; likewise, some people may require a dose or experience a side effect that is not described herein. Drugs and medical devices are discussed that may have limited availability controlled by the Food and Drug Administration (FDA) for use only in a research study or clinical trial. Research, clinical practice, and government regulations often change the accepted standard in this field. When consideration is being given to use of any drug in the clinical setting, the healthcare provider or reader is responsible for determining FDA status of the drug, reading the package insert, and reviewing prescribing information for the most up-to-date recommendations on dose, precautions, and contraindications, and determining the appropriate usage for the product. This is especially important in the case of drugs that are new or seldom used.

Production Credits
Executive Publisher: Christopher Davis
Editorial Assistant: Sara Cameron
Production Editor: Daniel Stone
Manufacturing and Inventory Control Supervisor: Amy Bacus
Senior Marketing Manager: Barb Bartoszek
Composition: Glyph International
Printing and Binding: Malloy, Inc.

Cover Credits
Cover Design: Colleen Lamy
Cover Printing: Malloy, Inc.
Cover Images: Top Left: © Photodisc; Bottom Left: © Photodisc; Right: © Enigmatico/Dreamstime.com.

Library of Congress Cataloging-in-Publication Data
Dizon, Don S.
    100 questions & answers about uterine cancer / Don S. Dizon, Linda R. Duska.
        p. cm.
    Includes index.
    ISBN 978-0-7637-7658-9 (alk. paper)
    1. Cervix uteri—Cancer—Popular works. 2. Cervix uteri—Cancer—Miscellanea. I. Title. II. Title: One hundred questions and answers about cervical cancer.
    RC280.U8D595 2011
    616.99'466—dc22
                                                2010006911
6048

Printed in the United States of America
14 13 12 11 10   10 9 8 7 6 5 4 3 2 1

This book is dedicated to the folks at The Program in Women's Oncology—superb clinicians, mid-level providers, nurses, social workers, integrative care specialists, and assistants, all dedicated to the care of women with cancer. Without them I would not have had the opportunities in my own career. You have helped me develop as a clinician and as a person, and for that I will be eternally grateful.

This is also dedicated to the patients who have allowed me into their lives at this very sensitive time. Living with cancer, its diagnosis, and its treatments is a task that only you can perform, and I have been struck by the sheer strength and determination that women diagnosed with uterine cancer bring to this fight. You are my inspiration to continue in this field.

This book is, last but not least, dedicated to my own family: my partner Henry, my daughters Isabelle and Sophia, and my son, Harrison; my parents, Modesto and Millonita; and my sisters, Michelle, Maerica, Precy, and Marie. You have always lent me your support—sharing in my pride, being there when I fall. I am able to accomplish all that I can because I know you will be there.

Finally, it is again dedicated to my family at Jones and Bartlett. The show of support in this partnership has been one of the gifts I have received in this academic career. Thank you.

Don S. Dizon, MD, FACP

As a practicing gynecologic oncologist, I see women with endometrial cancer more than any other gynecologic cancer. Most of these cancers are curable with surgery alone, or surgery plus vaginal radiation. Many of these women can be cured by simply removing their uterus. In recent years I have incorporated minimally invasive surgical techniques in my practice, allowing me to treat women with tiny incisions and short hospital stays. This, for me, is a very satisfying experience as endometrial cancer is one of the few cancers I treat that is so often cured. But however straightforward it is for me to treat these patients, it is a challenge for each new woman I meet with this diagnosis to come to grips with the fact that she has cancer. *Cancer*, after all, is a scary word (as is *surgery*!). My patients' courage serves as inspiration for me each and every day.

For each woman, we as care providers try to give as much education about the disease and the treatment involved; for each woman, we try to make the surgical experience as gentle as possible. And for each woman who entrusts her life and her body to me in the operating room, I am profoundly in awe of her bravery, her trust in my surgical skill, and her faith. I thank all of those women who have allowed me to be a part of their care and their "cancer journey." I hope that this book will help all women with endometrial cancer understand this disease a little bit better. Knowledge is power: we can treat and, in many cases, cure this cancer.

I dedicate my effort in this book to these women of courage, as well as the many special teachers and colleagues I have had the privilege to work with in the care of gynecologic cancers, both at the Cancer Center at the University of Virginia and the Gillette Center for Women's Cancers at the Massachusetts General Hospital. I am also very grateful to Don Dizon for asking me to be a part of this project, and for serving as mentor and friend for so many years.

Finally, I thank my family, without whose support I could never have completed the years of training required, and who always understand when I am in the operating room and late for dinner. Thank you Chris, Sarah, Jessica, Jacob, and Samuel; your love and support of my work for women with gynecologic cancer means more than you will ever know.

Linda R. Duska, MD

Contents

The fight against cancer happens in multiple ways. The surgeon removes the tumor, the medical oncologist prescribes chemotherapy, and the radiation oncologist prescribes radiotherapy. Yet it is the patient who must ask the questions and find the answers, and in the end, it is she who must have the surgery, the chemotherapy, and the radiation, and then deal with the side effects and consequences of being a cancer survivor.

In the shock of a new diagnosis, and the urgency to begin treatment, it is not uncommon that a woman gets halfway through the treatment and ponders, "what is happening," or "why am I going through this?" Even as providers strive to provide information that is accurate and timely, it is easy for us to fall back into the language of our peers, the "med-speak" that defines our careers, that provides the lexicon of our journals. I think, unfortunately, we often resort to med-speak in our explanations and even the best communicators among us can find ourselves in this predicament.

Yet, cancer is not a game; it is serious life-threatening illness. Uterine cancer is no exception. It has struck me that the resources for women with uterine cancer, though, are fairly sparse. Too often, women with uterine cancer resort to the literature applicable to women with ovarian cancer and, while this may be appropriate, there are differences in the management that make the extrapolation not quite fit.

As a result, Dr. Duska and I present *100 Questions & Answers About Uterine Cancer*. It is intended to be a guide for women diagnosed with uterine cancer, whether that be epithelial adenocarcinoma, uterine sarcoma, or gestational trophoblast disease. Some sections will be applicable only to some patients; others will have universal applicability. Some sections present questions that are difficult to raise and answers that are difficult to hear, but this book is intended to be a resource for all women with uterine cancer, no matter where they are in their own specific state of diagnosis, treatment, or follow-up.

More important than the information presented by the clinician's view, Dr. Duska and I were thrilled to have the participation of Joan Taylor, a cancer survivor herself. Her reflections on the questions posed provide the much-needed experience of one who has, and is, fighting that battle, on the front lines, as it were.

We hope we are addressing a critical need for women with uterine cancer. I would like to extend my deepest appreciation to Linda and to Joan for joining me in this collaboration. It represents a unique interdisciplinary view on the issues faced by women with uterine cancer, and we hope that our efforts will raise the level of awareness of your options and the current state of the science for that woman with uterine cancer and her family.

Don S. Dizon, MD, FACP

It is a privilege to have been asked to add my commentary to this book. Each of our cancer experiences stays individualized, but perhaps some of my thoughts will help one of you reading this book.

My cancer falls into the "none of the above" category. I do not show any of the "normal" risk factors and the cancer has spread in an atypical way. So the good news that my cancer was level 1 was turned around with a stage IIIC diagnosis. I am receiving the full range of available treatments—a sandwich approach of three sessions of chemotherapy followed by IMRT radiation and then brachytherapy followed by another three sessions of chemo. It is a long road but one willingly taken to reap the benefits of a long life.

I am very blessed to have friends who have stepped into the role of family. I would like to thank those special people for their support, love, and the food they so graciously are providing.

I have to thank my employer for the wonderful insurance that he provides. It means one less worry on this new road of my life.

I would like to dedicate this to those who are the "will" and the "way." My family members who, though far away, are the reason I'll be alive in thirty years. I have their love and energy with me every single day. They are the light of my life . . . my will to continued long life.

I am so fortunate to have a wonderful team of doctors, nurses, and their excellent staff who are my way to health and survivorship. It all starts with Dr. Pierre Manzo, my primary care physician; Dr. Michael Muto, my surgeon, Dr. Susana Campos and Dr. Akila Viswanathan, all at Dana-Farber Cancer Institute; and finally Dr. Don Dizon and Dr. M. Yakub Puthawala, here in Providence.

Joan Taylor

PART ONE

The Basics

Where is the uterus?

What are the types of uterine cancer?

What are the symptoms of uterine cancer?

More . . .

1. What is a tumor? What does benign mean? What does malignant mean?

A tumor is a growth that occurs in or on any part of the body. It comes from French, and means "an abnormal swelling of tissue." However, a tumor is more than just being swollen. It is made up of an abnormal collection of cells, but while a tumor is not normal, it is also not synonymous with cancer. Tumors can be non-threatening to your health (**benign**). A tumor can be a precancerous condition—which would require removing it, or it can be cancerous (**malignant**). Only by taking a piece of it (**biopsy**) or by removing it completely (**excision**) and then sending it to the lab for analysis by specially trained physicians (pathologists) can one be sure what category any tumor is in.

Benign tumors do not spread and usually can be left alone. However, they can also be quite large and, due to their size, can create symptoms worrisome for a more aggressive tumor. In such cases, they would still need to be removed. Once removed, benign tumors also will not warrant further treatment beyond surgery.

Malignant tumors are cancer. They can grow, spread, and can kill. These tumors are more urgently taken to surgery and may need to be treated after surgery.

2. What is cancer?

Cancer is the end product of cells that no longer follow the usual order of cell growth, division, and death. Instead, these cells divide uncontrollably, and grow out of control. In addition, these cells do not respect the normal borders between tissues. Instead they travel outside of their usual places, otherwise known as **metastasis**, or else grow beyond their own borders, also called **invasion**.

Benign
Non-threatening, non-cancerous.

Malignant
Cancerous. A growth with a tendency to invade and destroy nearby tissue and spread to other parts of the body.

Biopsy
Taking a piece of a tumor to determine whether it is malignant or benign.

Excision
Surgical removal of tissue.

Cancer
The end product of cells that no longer follow the usual order of cell growth, division, and death.

Metastasis
The spreading of a disease (especially cancer) to another part of the body.

Invasion
Growth of cancer cells into the underlying normal tissue.

The processes of uncontrolled cell growth, invasion, and metastasis are all hallmarks of cancer.

When we were still developing, first as babies inside our mothers and continuing on while we were infants and children, our cells rapidly grew and divided. The end result was **differentiation**—it's what enabled a red blood cell to carry oxygen, an intestinal cell to absorb food, and an ovarian cell to produce hormones to make eggs. If cells are injured or get too old, they undergo a process called **apoptosis**, or programmed cell death. This is what keeps us healthy and all our organs operating normally. Some of our organs keep the ability to divide in order to replace dead and dying cells. These include the skin, gastrointestinal tract, hair follicles, and, to a large degree, the ovaries, which replace their surface after an egg is released.

Differentiation

Changes in the cells of developing infants that enable cells to perform different functions.

Apoptosis

Programmed cell death.

If a cell undergoes changes in its building blocks, called DNA, it can escape this tightly regulated life cycle. These DNA changes, also called **mutations**, can allow cells to keep growing and dividing. They no longer respond to your body's signals to stop dividing, and this process of unchecked cell division results in a mass of such cells, called a *tumor*. If a tumor cell breaks free from its origin (in this case, the ovarian cell within the ovary), it can travel through the bloodstream and land in another area of one's body far away (in the lung, for example) and start growing there; it is by definition *metastatic*. These two features—unchecked cell growth and the ability to metastasize—define cancer.

Mutation

Changes in cell DNA which can allow irregular cell growth and division.

It is most important to realize that cancer is a disease, but is not an automatic death sentence.

It is most important to realize that cancer is a disease, but is not an automatic death sentence. More and more people, in fact, are cured from or are living longer with cancer. It used to be a very deadly condition, due to the

3

lack of effective treatments and screening. Thankfully, we have come a long way and innovations in treatment have made cancer increasingly more curable, and definitely less deadly. More and more we are thinking of cancer as a chronic medical condition and cancer survivorship has become a new field of practice to meet the needs of those living with a cancer diagnosis.

Joan said:

The day the doctor's office called and told me the doctor (who did my D&C) would like to see me in the afternoon for a consultation, I knew my life was forever changed. The hope that I just had fibroids was a thing of the past. I called a friend who had just had a hysterectomy to get the name of her surgeon–I figured I would need it. I didn't want to hear I had cancer but I knew I had to be prepared for it.

However, I firmly believe my attitude truly determines the extent cancer will disrupt my life and my relationships.

3. Is cancer contagious?

Cancer is not something that you can catch. It is not passed on from one person to another like the common cold or the flu, and it is not something that you can get from eating tainted food, like the bacteria E. coli (which causes infectious diarrhea). That is to say, cancer is not an infectious disease and is not contagious. Sometimes cancers will happen within a certain area or community, sometimes called a cancer cluster. In these cases, however, it is usually because a common poison or environmental factor is present that caused people living close together to all develop cancer.

In other situations, the presence of cancer in your father or mother may mean that cancer is passed on in families.

These cases are usually due to a genetic mutation, but these happen only in a minority of cases of cancer.

Some cancers are associated with a viral infection, like the human papillomavirus (HPV). HPV is associated with cervical, vulvar, and vaginal cancers, and is transmitted by sexual contact. However, not all women with HPV develop cancer and not all cancers are traceable to HPV. **Endometrial cancer** is not associated with HPV.

Endometrial Cancer
Cancer of the uterine lining.

4. Where is the uterus?

The ovaries, fallopian tubes, and uterus make up a woman's internal female reproductive organs and lie deep in the pelvis where they are connected to one another. The uterus attaches to the vagina at the cervix and is linked to the ovaries by the fallopian tubes.

The uterus responds to hormone levels and, in younger women, these responses lead to menstruation. The uterus is also connected by the fallopian tubes to the ovaries, and when an egg is released from the ovary, it travels via the fallopian tube into the uterus. A sperm meets an egg (fertilization) within the uterus. Embryos grow into babies inside of the uterus in a normal pregnancy.

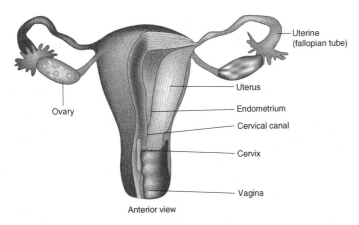

Anterior view

Figure 1   Female Reproductive Organs

5. What is the endometrium? Where exactly is it and what is its normal purpose?

There are two layers that make up the uterus: the **endometrium** and the **myometrium**. The endometrium lines the uterus and it becomes thicker when a woman's ovaries are producing estrogen. The myometrium is the muscular layer of the uterus and lies behind the endometrium.

The thickening of the endometrium is what makes it possible for the female body to support the growth of a baby. This thickening is caused by the hormone estrogen. After ovulation, the ovary produces another hormone, progesterone, which is intended to support the pregnancy. If pregnancy does not occur, the ovary will stop making progesterone causing the endometrial lining to slough off. The shedding of the endometrial lining is called menstruation, and happens monthly in the premenopausal woman. Women taking estrogen for hot flashes or for birth control will develop thickening of their endometrium. Without a break from the estrogen, this thickness can become abnormal and develop into cancer. This is why it's important to use progesterone or else have a limit on the time one's body sees estrogen.

6. What is a fibroid? Can it become a uterine cancer?

A **fibroid** is a muscular tumor of the uterus and develops from the wall of the uterus and can develop into the uterine cavity (called a **submucosal fibroid**), within the wall of the uterus (called an **intramural fibroid**), or outside of the uterus (called a **subserosal fibroid**). They can even develop as an outpouching connected to the uterus by a stalk, much like a mushroom (called a **pedunculated fibroid**). The medical term for it is a **leiomyoma**

Endometrium

Lining of the uterus which becomes thicker when a woman's ovaries are producing estrogen.

Myometrium

The muscular layer of the uterus that lies behind the endometrium.

Fibroid

A muscular tumor that develops from the wall of the uterus and can develop into the uterine cavity (called a submucosal fibroid), within the wall of the uterus (called an intramural fibroid), or outside of the uterus (subserosal fibroid).

Leiomyoma

Benign tumor of smooth muscle, usually the uterus. Also referred to as myoma.

or myoma. They commonly occur, particularly in a woman's 30s or 40s, and usually shrink down after she reaches menopause. Risks for developing fibroids include a positive family history of them, African American race, obesity, and a diet rich in red meat. Fibroids typically don't bother women, but if they are large can cause pain, particularly during periods. Large fibroids can also complicate fertility and the normal course of pregnancy. Other symptoms include heavy menstrual periods, fullness in the pelvis, abdominal enlargement, pain during intercourse, and low back pain.

Fibroids, by definition, are not cancer and we do not think they can develop into a cancer. However, there is a type of muscular cancer of the uterus, called a **leiomyosarcoma**, which can sometimes present as a previously diagnosed fibroid that appears to grow far too quickly.

7. How do you screen for uterine cancer?

There is no screening system for uterine cancer, though sometimes a **Pap smear**, which is used to screen for cervical cancer, will detect cancer cells coming from the uterus. The Pap test is a procedure done during a pelvic examination and is performed at both gynecology and primary care physicians' offices. It involves a speculum exam, which is how your doctor can see the cervix. Once it is seen, a spatula or a brush is used to scrape the cervix surface and the cervical os, which is the mouth or opening of the cervix. The scrapings can then be sent to the lab for analysis. Most Pap tests today are performed using liquid-based methods because additional tests can be performed on the sample collected from the cervix. The Thin Prep® Pap test is the only FDA-approved liquid-based Pap test for the detection of HPV, Gonorrhea, and Chlamydia out of the vial.

Fibroids, by definition, are not cancer and we do not think they can develop into a cancer.

The Basics

Leiomyosarcoma

A type of muscular cancer of the uterus, which can sometimes present as a previously diagnosed fibroid that appears to grow far too quickly.

Pap smear or Pap test

A procedure done during a pelvic examination at both gynecology and primary care physicians' offices. It involves a speculum exam which is how your doctor can see the cervix.

Pap tests today are performed using liquid-based methods because additional tests can be performed on the sample collected from the cervix.

The Thin Prep® Pap test has also been shown to better detect abnormalities involving the glands of the cervix, as compared to the conventional Pap smear. This is important because one form of cervical cancer involving the glands, called **adenocarcinoma**, is on the rise in the United States today, particularly in younger women. Using this technology, pathologists can sometimes pick up abnormal cells coming from higher up the reproductive system and can sometimes detect uterine adenocarcinomas.

Adenocarcinoma
A form of cancer that arises from the glands.

It is important to remember that the Pap smear is not intended to screen for endometrial cancer. A woman can have a normal Pap smear and still have endometrial cancer.

Fortunately, most women will present with symptoms early on in the disease. Other symptoms are discussed in Question 10.

8. How big of a problem is uterine cancer?

Each year, more than 40,000 women are diagnosed with uterine cancer and 7,400 women die of the disease in the United States. The majority of these cases are adenocarcinomas. Worldwide it affects almost 200,000 women each year, with 50,000 deaths due to uterine cancer.

9. What are the types of uterine cancer?

The uterus can give rise to different cancers. The most common is a glandular tumor that starts in the endometrium, called endometrial adenocarcinoma. Sometimes a distinction is made between two types of adenocarcinoma. Type I endometrial cancers are associated with excessive estrogen exposure, tend to present with uterine bleeding, and are seen in women with a family history of either colon or uterine cancers. Type II cancers, on the other hand, tend to present without any signs of problems and are of a more aggressive nature. We will touch on these more in Question 16.

Sarcomas can also arise from the uterus: they can arise from the muscle cells, the surrounding stromal cells, or the endometrium itself. The most common sarcomas are leiomyosarcoma, endometrial stromal sarcoma, and carcinosarcoma. During a normal pregnancy, the uterine placenta feeds the growing baby. However, in rare cases the placenta itself can be cancerous, giving rise to **gestational trophoblast neoplasia (GTN)**. In the first part of the book we will concentrate on uterine adenocarcinoma, but we will also touch on the other tumors of the uterus as well.

Gestational trophoblast neoplasia (GTN)

A very rare group of tumors that can grow from cells inside a woman's uterus.

10. What are the symptoms of uterine cancer?

As discussed in Question 7, the usual symptom of the most common type of uterine cancer is abnormal or heavy bleeding. This bleeding may be red blood like a menstrual period, or may be very scant. Some women describe their symptoms as "staining" and some experience only a brown discharge on their underpants or mini-pad. If a post-menopausal woman experiences these symptoms, she should go to her gynecologist. In the pre-menopause, a woman might experience more heavy menses or bleeding between periods as a symptom of endometrial cancer. However, other symptoms that may be present include the development of a blood-tinged vaginal discharge, pain with sex, pain with making urine, abdominal swelling (or bloating), or constipation. Persisting symptoms should be brought to the attention of your doctor as soon as possible. These symptoms are generally seen in adenocarcinomas of the uterus. Sometimes, the sarcomas will present with bloating or a rapidly growing pelvic mass.

The usual symptom of the most common type of uterine cancer is abnormal or heavy bleeding.

Women with a rare type of uterine cancer called gestational trophoblast neoplasia (GTN) will usually have a positive pregnancy test as their first sign of a problem. When there is a lack of a fetus by an ultrasound or serial human chorionic gonadotropin (hCG) blood levels are abnormally increasing, GTN must be ruled out.

We will focus most of this book on adenocarcinomas of the uterus. However, Questions 48–54 will specifically deal with sarcomas and Questions 55–64 will speak about GTN.

Joan said:

I only experienced a slight vaginal discharge. I am post menopausal so it wasn't anything "normal" and I knew I had to have it checked out. I had no other indications of something going on but I knew I had to have it checked out promptly.

PART TWO

Risk Factors

Are there risk factors for uterine cancer?

How can uterine cancer run in families?

Can medications cause uterine cancer?

More . . .

11. Are there risk factors for uterine cancer?

The risk factors for uterine adenocarcinomas (Type I) are associated with excessive estrogen stimulation. Women who are obese, have polycystic ovarian syndrome, or take unopposed estrogen replacement (as seen with drugs like tamoxifen or estrogen-only hormone replacement treatment) are at risk. Other risk factors include diabetes mellitus and family history of colon and/or uterine cancer, which may point to an inherited syndrome that will increase your risk, called **hereditary non-polyposis colorectal cancer syndrome (HNPCC)**.

One of the biggest contributing risk factors for uterine cancer is obesity. Obesity is defined as a Body-Mass Index (also called BMI) of greater than 30. The fat tissue, called **adipose**, is able to store high levels of hormones that can be converted to estrogen and stimulate the endometrium to create endometrial cancer. Obese women can decrease their risk of developing endometrial cancer by modifying their lifestyle to normalize their BMI.

Joan said:

I don't meet any of the normally listed risk factors. I have been a little overweight but never obese and there is no family history for inheritance. It is a puzzle to me but I certainly don't dwell on the "why me" in life. Knowing I cannot pass it to my children lets me leave the why's behind.

12. How can uterine cancer run in families?

Uterine cancers can occur in families due to the passage of a DNA mutation that causes an abnormality in the genes that helps them remain normal. The mutation that runs in some families that can increase this risk

Hereditary non-polyposis colcorectal cancer syndrome (HNPCC)

An inherited syndrome that will increase your risk of uterine cancer.

One of the biggest contributing risk factors for uterine cancer is obesity.

Adipose

The fat tissue, which is able to store high levels of hormones that can be converted to estrogen and stimulate the endometrium to create endometrial cancer.

causes **microsatellite instability (MSI)**. The hallmark of this is the syndrome of HNPCC, in which families will have affected members not only with uterine cancer, but also with colon cancers. Unfortunately, the passing of this mutation is not something that can be prevented now, though work in the field of reproduction may change this in the future by allowing the studying of fertilized eggs (or embryos) and identifying normal versus abnormal embryos that harbor this mutation. By not implanting those that have the mutation, one can have a child with no increased risk of HNPCC. This is called **preimplantation genetic analysis**, but the field is still in development.

Microsatellite instability (MSI)
Predisposition to certain cancers that runs in some families caused by passage of a DNA mutation.

Preimplantation genetic analysis
The study of fertilized eggs (or embryos) to identify normal versus abnormal embryos.

Risk Factors

13. I had heard that women with breast cancer can get uterine cancer. Is that true?

Women who are taking a selective estrogen blocker like Tamoxifen can indeed get uterine cancer. This happens because Tamoxifen will specifically block estrogen from seeing breast tissue, but not anywhere else. That is, it acts selectively when blocking the estrogen receptor. This means that other tissue, like bones and the uterus, perceive Tamoxifen as an estrogen, and in the uterus, it can cause the lining to build up. Since there is no period of withdrawal from this estrogenic stimulation, the buildup can persist and can predispose to the development of uterine cancer. Frequently, the primary sign of a problem when on Tamoxifen is abnormal uterine bleeding. If this happens, you should see your doctor immediately. The work-up usually entails an ultrasound of the uterus to see if thickening is present (often referred to as the endometrial stripe). The work-up also calls for a tissue analysis, often obtained from an endometrial curettage or biopsy. Beyond this, women who have had breast cancer can develop uterine cancer as part of a genetic

Women who are taking a selective estrogen blocker like Tamoxifen can indeed get uterine cancer.

13

risk. These cancers are a part of the HNPCC syndrome noted in Question 12.

It is important to note that most women who take Tamoxifen will not develop endometrial cancer. In the early very large studies of Tamoxifen and women with breast cancer, the women who developed endometrial cancer developed it very early, in the first 12 months of taking Tamoxifen. This might suggest that these women had an underlying abnormality of their endometrium that was not diagnosed before they started Tamoxifen. If you are going to take Tamoxifen it is important to see your gynecologist regularly and report any abnormal vaginal bleeding you might be having before you start the Tamoxifen or while you are taking it.

14. Can medications cause uterine cancer?

Yes, particularly estrogen-containing compounds. In addition to Tamoxifen, using estrogen replacement therapy can increase the risk of uterine cancer. This is why, if used, it is given with progesterone, which is another female hormone that usually helps to support a pregnancy. Progesterone is included in combined hormonal preparations and is required to reduce the risk of uterine cancer in susceptible women. Beyond hormonally-acting agents, there are no other medications linked with the diagnosis of uterine cancer.

PART THREE

Uterine Epithelial Cancer

Are there different classifications of tumors?
How are they different?

What is the difference between a computed
tomography (CT) and magnetic resonance imaging
(MRI) in working up uterine cancer?

What is tumor "stage"? How is uterine cancer staged?

More . . .

15. What does it mean to have an endometrial adenocarcinoma?

As we discussed, endometrial adenocarcinomas arise from the lining of the endometrium, and hence are also termed epithelial cancers. The specific type of adeno-carcinoma is diagnosed by the pathologist, based on what the cells look like when seen under a microscope. The most common of the epithelial adenocarcinomas is called endometrioid adenocarcinoma. Other types of uterine adenocarcinomas are:

- Papillary
- Secretory
- Ciliated cell
- Adenocarcinoma with squamous differentiation
- Mucinous
- Clear cell

When the cells under the microscope are so abnormal that they do not look like any of those listed above, the pathologist may refer to it as an "Undifferentiated" adenocarcinoma.

Joan said:

It means a whole new vocabulary and a whole new world to Google (with care in selecting the sites you visit). I asked my surgeon the first time I met him which websites he would recommend and stuck to those and added the cancer center he is associated with. You learn it means you are one of the lucky ones—it is the best of the bad possibilities.

16. Are there different classifications of tumors? How are they different?

In addition to distinguishing them by histology, doctors can think of them as two "types" called Type I and Type II.

Type I endometrial cancer is caused by an excess of the hormone estrogen. This excess can be caused by taking unopposed estrogen (estrogen without progesterone), but it can also be caused by obesity because fat cells store hormones that the body converts into estrogen. Women who develop Type I endometrial cancer are often post menopausal (in their sixth decade) and obese. They may suffer from gall bladder disease and have diabetes.

Type I cancers are usually endometrioid type and are usually grade I, or well differentiated. They are often associated with a specific genetic mutation involving a loss of PTEN, which can be checked in a lab under the microscope. Type I cancers also are often associated with a condition of the endometrium called **complex atypical hyperplasia**, which is thought to be a precursor lesion for endometrioid adenocarcinoma of the endometrium.

Type II cancers, on the other hand, are not associated with excess estrogen, and are usually more aggressive. They occur in women who are older, in their seventh decade and above, and are often high grade, or papillary serous. These cancers have a worse prognosis than Type I cancers and often stain under the microscope for a marker called p53. They can be associated with **endometrial intraepithelial neoplasia**, also called EIN, which is thought to be a precursor lesion for uterine serous papillary carcinoma.

17. How do you diagnose uterine carcinoma?

Fortunately endometrial cancer is usually diagnosed early; approximately 80% of cases are diagnosed as stage I, or confined to the uterus, also called the corpus. This is because most women have symptoms early in

Uterine Epithelial Cancer

Type I endometrial cancer

Caused by an excess of the hormone estrogen.

Complex atypical hyperplasia

A condition of the endometrium which is thought to be a precursor lesion for endometrioid adenocarcinoma.

Type II cancers

These are not associated with excess estrogen, and are usually more aggressive.

Endometrial intraepithelial neoplasia (EIN)

Condition thought to be a precursor lesion for uterine serous papillary carcinoma.

The most common symptom of endometrial cancer is post-menopausal bleeding.

Pipelle biopsy

Biopsy performed in the physician's office with a soft plastic straw called a pipelle.

D&C

D&C stands for dilatation and curettage. In this procedure the surgeon will dilate, or open, the cervix in order to perform a curettage, or scraping, of the uterine cavity.

Hysteroscopy

A tool used to help direct the curettage in which a fiber-optic scope is used to look inside the uterus.

the course of the disease that bring them to the doctor. The most common symptom of endometrial cancer is post-menopausal bleeding.

The doctor will diagnose endometrial cancer by performing a biopsy of the endometrium. This biopsy can be performed in one of two ways. The first way is to perform a biopsy in the office with a soft plastic straw called a **"pipelle" biopsy**. Most of the time, this biopsy can be performed with minimal discomfort to the patient at the time of an office visit.

Sometimes an office biopsy either cannot be performed or does not result in a diagnosis. In that case, a diagnosis can be made with a D&C in the operating room. **D&C** stands for dilatation and curettage. In this procedure the surgeon will dilate, or open, the cervix in order to perform a curettage, or scraping, of the uterine cavity. This procedure will allow the endometrium to be collected and sent to pathology for diagnosis. Sometimes a tool called **hysteroscopy** is also used to help direct the curettage. A fiber-optic scope is used to look inside the uterus so the surgeon can be sure the abnormal area of endometrium is correctly sampled.

18. Are there blood tests that can be used to screen for or diagnose uterine cancer?

Unfortunately, there are no blood tests that can be done to screen for or diagnose uterine cancer. A blood test used in ovarian cancer that checks for CA-125 can sometimes be elevated in advanced uterine cancer, Grade 3, or serous type adenocarcinomas, but for the most part, it is not a useful test to try to pick up uterine cancer earlier.

19. I had an ultrasound for uterine cancer. What exactly are they looking for?

Ultrasound can be used to measure something called the endometrial stripe. By doing this measurement, the doctor can assess if there is an abnormality in the endometrium. A thick endometrial stripe is not normal in a post-menopausal woman, but is not always diagnostic of endometrial cancer. For example, an endometrial polyp, which is often benign, can make the endometrial stripe look thick on ultrasound. Sometimes the doctor will use saline infusion along with the ultrasound to help assess whether or not there is a polyp in the endometrial cavity.

Ultrasound is a painless test that is not as expensive as other tests such as MRI or CT scan. Usually the doctor will order both a transabdominal and transvaginal ultrasound. For the transvaginal part of the ultrasound, the technician will ask the woman to insert the ultrasound probe into her vagina. The transvaginal part of the study is often the most useful for evaluating the ovaries and the endometrial stripe, particularly in women who are overweight. While it might be a little uncomfortable and is embarrassing for some women, it is not usually painful.

If a saline injection into the uterus is used, for example to diagnose a polyp, there can be some cramping as the saline is injected into the endometrial cavity.

Ultrasound can also be used to look at the ovaries and fallopian tubes to be sure they are normal. Rarely, endometrial cancer can spread to the tubes and ovaries.

20. What are lymph nodes and are they important in diagnosis?

Lymph nodes are bean sized organs that are part of the immune system and are present throughout the body. There are lymph nodes lining all of the big arteries and veins in the abdomen and pelvis. When it spreads, endometrial cancer can spread to the lymph nodes; though this is uncommon in Type I cancers, it is more common in Type II cancers.

In order to determine whether lymph nodes are involved with cancer, they must be removed surgically and looked at under the microscope. This can be done at the time of hysterectomy for endometrial cancer. **Gynecologic Oncologists** are surgeons who can perform this type of "staging" surgery for patients with endometrial cancer. Not all patients with endometrial cancer need to have their lymph nodes removed. Patients with grade I cancers that invade less than half of the uterine muscle probably do not have to have their lymph nodes removed because the risk of metastasis to the lymph nodes is very low.

For higher risk endometrial cancers, for example Type II cancers, the status of the lymph nodes is very important in making decisions about more treatment after surgery. If a patient is found to have positive lymph nodes, her doctor may recommend chemotherapy or radiation treatment to prevent future cancer recurrence.

If a patient is found to have positive lymph nodes, her doctor may recommend chemotherapy or radiation treatment to prevent future cancer recurrence.

While there are some risks associated with removing the lymph nodes in the pelvis, these are fortunately rare. They include increased bleeding at the time of the surgery, risk of damage to the arteries or veins in the pelvis, or damage to nerves that run along with the lymph nodes.

In particular, the genitofemoral nerve can be damaged during removal of pelvic lymph nodes. If this occurs, the woman might have a small numb patch on the front of her thigh; there will be no effect on leg strength or mobility.

After a lymph node dissection, a woman may experience swelling in her feet or legs. This is called lymphedema and is fortunately not very common. There can also be a collection of fluid in the area of the lymph node removal called a "lymphocyst." These are often asymptomatic but sometimes need to be drained.

21. What is a PET scan? Are they good for diagnosis?

FDG-PET stands for **fluorodeoxyglucose positron emission test**. It is a radiologic study that uses information about the metabolism or activity of tumors to determine the extent a cancer has spread. A PET scan is done by labeling glucose (or sugar) molecule with a radioactive tag and then scanning for where these molecules show up in the body. Highly metabolic or active spots are suspicious for being cancerous, although there are areas, such as the kidney or bladder, that routinely show activity as well. Oftentimes, PET scans are combined with **computed tomography (CT)** to help give both a structural and functional assessment of a tumor. For instance, an area of activity on a PET scan appears as a blurry area on the outline of your body. Adding a CT scan allows your doctor to locate the area on a PET scan to see if there is a growth or tumor that corresponds to that activity. The role of PET scanning in endometrial cancer is not clear, as it is not a good test to determine how deeply involved an endometrial cancer is. It can determine if there are sites of activity outside of the pelvis, which is helpful

Fluorodeoxyglucose positron emission test (FDG-PET)

A radiologic study that uses information about the metabolism or activity of tumors to determine the extent a cancer has spread.

Computed tomography (CT)

Test which uses x-rays to build a picture and is sometimes administered in combination with a PET scan to help give both a structural and functional assessment of a tumor.

in making the treatment plan. PET scans can be done to see if your cancer has become metastatic or has recurred. There are ongoing studies looking at the role of PET scans in uterine cancer. Over time, it is likely to become a well-accepted and frequently performed test for women with cancer of the uterus suspected of having disease beyond the pelvis.

At the time of this writing, there is no indication to order a PET scan prior to surgery for endometrial cancer. Often just an ultrasound is done pre-operatively. Sometimes a CT scan of the abdomen and pelvis will be ordered to look for enlarged lymph nodes; this is particularly useful in Type II cancers, which are more likely to go to the lymph nodes.

22. What is the difference between a computed tomography (CT) and magnetic resonance imaging (MRI) in working up uterine cancer?

Magnetic resonance imaging (MRI)

MRI uses radio waves traveling through a magnetic field to significantly make out what is being imaged (that is, what is normal versus abnormal and how they relate to each other).

A CT scan uses x-rays to build a picture. To make contrasts between blood vessels, lymph nodes, and normal, typically an iodine-based dye is used (to help light up vessels) and barium contrast is drunk (to help outline the stomach, small intestines, and colon). In these ways, CT scans can distinguish between flesh, bone, and blood vessels. It is a good way to evaluate a tumor's size and whether or not there is evidence of spread, and it is frequently used to stage endometrial cancer.

MRI stands for magnetic resonance imaging. MRI uses radio waves traveling through a magnetic field. By using contrast agents, it can significantly make out what is being imaged (that is, what is normal versus abnormal and how they relate to each other). In women with endometrial cancer, it is a great test to determine if a uterine cancer is superficial (meaning, it is arising within the endometrium) or deeply invasive (meaning it is so big it involves the deeper muscular layers of the uterus or even involves structures outside of the uterus). MRIs cannot be done if patients are too obese, have metal in their body, or are claustrophobic as it requires one to sit or lie down in a container that is required to be closed.

23. What is a tumor "grade"?

The **grade** is a way to describe what cancer cells look like under the microscope and to the degree they appear abnormal. The degree of changes seen in the cells tells the pathologist how abnormal cancer cells are. Grade is defined as I, II, or III. Grade I cancers are otherwise known as "well-differentiated" and appear very similar to normal cells. Their presence outside of the normal boundaries would define them as cancer. As cancers look increasingly abnormal, the grade gets higher. Thus, grade II cancers are moderately differentiated and grade III cancers are poorly differentiated.

24. What is tumor "stage"? How is uterine cancer staged?

The **stage of cancer** refers to how much of the body is involved at the time of diagnosis. In general, one can break down the stages into those without spread outside of the organ in which they start (stage I) and those that have spread locally (stages II, III) or to distant sites (metastases) (stage IV). The system for staging uterine cancer is set by the International Federation of Gynecology and Obstetrics (FIGO).

Uterine Epithelial Cancer

Grade

A term used to describe what cancer cells look like under the microscope and the degree to which they appear abnormal.

As cancers look increasingly abnormal, the grade gets higher. Thus, grade II cancers are moderately differentiated and grade III cancers are poorly differentiated.

Stage of cancer

Refers to how much of the body is involved at the time of diagnosis.

As applied to uterine cancer, its earliest is Stage I, when it is confined solely to the uterus. In Stage II, there is spread below the uterus into the cervix. In Stage III, the cancer has moved to lymph nodes, the vagina, or into the pelvis where the ovaries live. In Stage IV, there is either locally advanced disease involving the bladder or bowel wall or, at its most extensive, it has spread beyond the pelvis, to the fatty apron surrounding the bowels (the **omentum**), liver, or lungs. Involvement of the lymph nodes where the thigh meets the hip (the inguinal area) also connotes Stage IV disease. These are summarized in Table 1.

Omentum

The fatty apron surrounding the bowels.

Table 1   Staging of Endometrial Cancer

For all stages, must specify tumor grade	
Stage I: Tumor confined to the uterine corpus	
IA	No or less than half myometrial invasion
IB	Invasion equal to or more than half of the myometrium
Stage II: Tumor invades cervical stroma, but does not extend beyond the uterus	
Stage III: Local and/or regional spread of the tumor	
IIIA	Tumor invades the serosa of the uterine corpus and/or ovaries
IIIB	Vaginal and/or parametrial involvement
IIIC	Metastases to pelvic and/or paraaortic lymph nodes
IIIC1	Positive pelvic nodes
IIIC2	Positive para-aortic lymph nodes ± positive pelvic lymph nodes
Stage IV: Tumor invades bladder and/or bowel mucosa, and/or distant metastases	
IVA	Tumor invasion of bladder and/or bowel mucosa
IVB	Distant metastases, including intra-abdominal metastases and/or inguinal lymph nodes

25. How does uterine cancer spread?

Cancer can spread in three ways: by extending into surrounding tissue; by passing through the blood supply, a process called **hematogenous dissemination**; or by traveling in the **lymphatic system**, the "cleaning system" of the body, in a process termed *lymphatic spread*. Uterine cancer can spread in all of these ways. Knowing the ways in which cancers spread is important, because such knowledge often is used to decide what type of surgery is necessary and what other types of treatment are necessary (such as the use of chemotherapy and the number of cycles needed).

Hematogenous dissemination

Process in which cancer spreads by passing through the blood supply.

Lymphatic system

The "cleaning system" of the body.

Uterine Epithelial Cancer

PART FOUR

Treatment of Epithelial Cancers of the Uterus

Is there any way to treat uterine cancers that doesn't require surgery?

Do I need to have my ovaries removed? My cervix?

What kind of chemotherapy is used to treat uterine cancer?

More . . .

26. Is there any way to treat uterine cancers that doesn't require surgery?

Surgery is the best treatment for endometrial cancer and results in the highest cure rates. Sometimes a woman cannot have surgery, usually because she is too medically ill to have general anesthesia, or because she has other problems that make surgery technically difficult, such as morbid obesity. In these cases there are other options.

A woman with a grade I cancer that appears to be confined to the endometrium (based on MRI most commonly) can be treated with hormones alone. This treatment does not always work, but can be successful in "reversing" the cancer in approximately 60% of cases. Most doctors use the hormone progesterone by mouth, but an IUD (intrauterine device) with progesterone in it can also be used. The woman must undergo sequential endometrial biopsies in order to be sure that the cancer has "reversed" and, after reversal, she must remain on lifetime progesterone. Progesterone has significant side effects, including weight gain, breast tenderness, and increased risk of blood clot.

Alternatively, the woman may be treated with radiation therapy. Usually intracavitary applicators (in the vagina) are used, along with whole pelvic radiation. A woman can be cured with radiation alone, but the cure rates are lower than they are for surgery or surgery plus radiation. There are also complications associated with radiation, including diarrhea, fatigue, and damage to bowel and bladder.

27. How do I decide by whom and where I should be treated?

Once the diagnosis of endometrial cancer has been made, you should see a Gynecologic Oncologist for your surgery if this is possible. Gynecologic Oncologists have the most experience with endometrial cancer. Unlike gynecologists, Gynecologic Oncologists can remove lymph nodes if indicated and understand the indications for lymph node removal. In addition, a Gynecologic Oncologist can counsel you post operatively about the need for more therapy after the hysterectomy and can appropriately provide post-treatment surveillance.

Gynecologic Oncologists are often experts in minimally invasive surgical techniques for treating endometrial cancer, including laparoscopy and robotic surgery (covered in Question 38).

Joan said:

I was not comfortable with the gynecologist I was referred to for my D&C. I was lucky to have a medical contact (doctor) through my work and he was able to refer me to a wonderful gynecological oncologist for my hysterectomy. Go to the best cancer center that is available to you. At the very least, get a second opinion. That second doctor will also enable you to have a contact for a second opinion when/if you need additional treatments such as radiation and/or chemotherapy.

If you aren't comfortable with your current doctor, CHANGE! And remember there is no question you cannot ask.

28. My surgeon recommends that I have my uterus removed. How do they do this?

The traditional method of removing the uterus for endometrial cancer is to remove it abdominally, through a vertical incision in the abdomen, called a **laparotomy**. This can sometimes also be accomplished through a transverse incision, or "bikini cut," depending on your

Laparotomy

An incision in the abdomen, through which the uterus is removed.

particular type of cancer and the shape of your abdomen. For endometrial cancer, the uterus, cervix, and both tubes and ovaries are removed.

Some surgeons can perform this surgery either with a laparoscope or a robotically assisted laparoscope. This sort of surgery allows for a shorter hospital stay and shorter recovery, and studies have shown that it gives the same result for curing the cancer. Not every woman will be a candidate for this "minimally invasive" kind of surgery.

Joan said:

I did a lot of research on selected websites—mostly so I would be a little more knowledgeable with the new vocabulary I would be hearing. I created a notebook from the beginning—starting with the different types of hysterectomies that are performed and the specifics of each one. Reading up enabled me to better understand the doctor's explanations and recommendations.

29. Can I have my surgery done vaginally?

A vaginal hysterectomy is a reasonable surgical choice for carefully selected patients. The standard approach still requires total hysterectomy and removal of the ovaries. For women who are very large or who have significant medical illnesses, a vaginal approach can minimize the risk of postoperative complications. When a vaginal approach is combined with laparoscopy, one can ensure a full surgical evaluation for endometrial cancer, but vaginal approaches by themselves should be restricted to women at risk from surgery and who have early-stage endometrial cancers. This is because the lymph nodes can't be removed at the time of a vaginal surgery.

A vaginal only approach is very limiting because it does not allow the surgeon to survey the abdomen and pelvis. In addition, not all gynecologists can remove ovaries through the vagina. The addition of the laparoscope allows both survey of the abdomen and removal of the ovaries.

30. Do I need to have my ovaries removed? My cervix?

As noted in Question 29, removal of the cervix and ovaries is required for complete surgical treatment of endometrial cancer. In young women, the ovaries may be spared, but the risk that cancer may be present there must be discussed in great detail. For women who may have their ovaries removed, fertility preservation strategies should be discussed beforehand, including the options of freezing eggs or embryos or even ovarian tissue preservation. For women with endometrial cancer, the cervix must be removed. It is part of the staging system of endometrial cancer and speaks to the high risk that it may be involved. It would be inappropriate to perform a hysterectomy but leave the cervix in place.

Endometrial cancer is not usually a disease of young women but sometimes women under 40 may develop endometrial cancer. These women might want to keep their ovaries for the purpose of keeping their hormones until menopause. We know that women who are under 40 who develop endometrial cancer are also at risk for developing an ovarian cancer later on (also called synchronous primary). If they elect to keep their ovaries, these women must be very carefully counseled about their risk of developing ovarian cancer and should consider having their ovaries removed when they reach menopause.

Endometrial cancer is not usually a disease of young women but sometimes women under 40 may develop endometrial cancer.

31. My surgeon mentioned removing my lymph nodes. What are they?

The lymph nodes are bean sized structures that are part of the immune system. Endometrial cancer can spread to the lymph nodes along the veins and arteries in the pelvis. Your surgeon can remove these lymph nodes in order to determine whether they are involved with cancer and to help make recommendations about the need for more therapy after surgery.

32. Do all women with uterine cancer need to have their lymph nodes removed?

Some Gynecologic Oncologists believe that it is important to remove all of the lymph nodes in the pelvis and along the aorta in all cases of endometrial cancer, but most agree that certain patients can avoid this procedure: women with grade 1 endometrioid tumors that are minimally invasive (less than halfway through) of the muscle of the uterus have a very low risk of lymph node involvement. Therefore the lymph nodes do not need to be removed.

Women whose pelvic lymph nodes are negative have a very low risk of having their para-aortic nodes be positive. This risk is probably less than 5%. Some gynecologic oncologists will, therefore, take out only the pelvic lymph nodes.

33. Are there side effects or long-term problems associated with removing your lymph nodes?

There are side effects associated with having lymph nodes removed. Lymph node removal makes the surgery take longer and can also result in a higher risk of bleeding during surgery. In the short term after surgery, some women can develop **lymphocysts**, or fluid filled pockets where the lymph nodes used to be. These can be asymptomatic, but sometimes a woman will have symptoms and the lymphocysts will need to be drained.

In the long term, some women will develop **lymphedema**, or swelling in their feet and lower legs, following a lymph node dissection. This occurs in about 5% of women who have this procedure done and seems to be worse if post-operative radiation therapy is required. Treatments for lymphedema include compression stockings and massage; in severe cases a pump may be used.

Joan said:

This was a big worry to me. Once in the lymphatic system, would the cancer just be everywhere? How long would it take to show up somewhere else? There are no specific answers—each is an individual case. I was lucky to have a medical oncologist and a radiation oncologist in Boston who referred me to Providence oncologists. Between them all, I knew I had the best doctors to call on and that was/is a great comfort to me. Again, websites gave me a heads up on possible side effects and I could ask intelligent questions of my doctors and know what to look out for in the future.

34. How does a surgeon decide whether to take the lymph nodes?

Most surgeons will remove lymph nodes for cancers that are high grade (grades 2 and 3), for cancers of all grades that are deeply invasive into the muscle, and for all papillary serous and clear cell cancers. That is because these cancers are at high risk for lymph node involvement. If you have evidence of ovarian involvement or enlarged lymph nodes, the lymph nodes should be removed.

Lymphocysts

A collection of fluid-filled pockets in the area of a lymph node removal.

Lymphedema

Swelling in the feet or legs that a woman may experience after a lymph node dissection.

Treatment of Epithelial Cancers of the Uterus

Beyond this, there are multiple ways a surgeon can determine if lymph nodes are involved in uterine cancer. The first is at the time of surgery—when the lymph nodes are removed at the time of the hysterectomy. The second method is by doing a biopsy with a needle. The health care provider performing the needle biopsy is usually aided by radiology. Using a CT scan machine, the needle can be guided to the suspicious area. The third technique is by PET/CT scan. In this combined scan, abnormal active areas are correlated with areas that are also enlarged, and if both are present in the lymph nodes in a woman with cancer, it is considered proof of metastatic disease. In such a case, your doctor may not even proceed to a biopsy or excision.

For grade 1 cancers, the surgeon may wait until the uterus has been removed to make a final decision about the lymph nodes. A "frozen section" of the uterus is obtained while you are asleep to assess how invasive into the muscle of the uterus your cancer is. If your cancer is more than halfway through the muscle of the uterus (the myometrium) then removal of the lymph nodes should be strongly considered.

35. If I didn't have my nodes removed, should I go back to the operating room?

If your cancer is an endometrioid cancer that is grade 1 or 2, is less than halfway through the muscle of the uterus, and does not show involvement of vascular spaces in the uterus, then your risk of lymph node involvement is very low and you probably will not need to go back to the operating room to have lymph nodes removed, but ultimately it will be up to your surgeon and you to make this decision.

If you have a high grade or deeply invasive cancer, then your risk of having lymph node involvement is high enough to warrant intervention. However, your doctor may recommend radiation to the lymph node areas without a return to the operating room if your risk is high enough. Your doctor may discuss going back to the operating room to remove lymph nodes with you if he or she believes you might be able to avoid radiation if your lymph nodes are negative, or if there is evidence of enlarged lymph nodes on CT scan.

Joan said:

I did have my pelvic lymph nodes removed at the time of my hysterectomy but not the para aortic nodes. It was something I made sure to talk about with my surgeon and also the oncologists handling my follow-up treatments. I was concerned how we would know if they were involved or not.

36. What is robotic surgery? Is this an option for me? What about laparoscopy?

Robotic surgery is a special kind of laparoscopic surgery in which robotic "arms" are attached to the laparoscopic instruments. The robot allows the surgeon to have more freedom of motion and also to see your operation in three dimensions, as opposed to two dimensions with laparoscopy. Both laparoscopy and robotic surgery are called "minimally invasive" because they do not require a large incision in the abdomen but instead use multiple small incisions through which "trocars" are placed. Your surgery is done by long instruments that go through these trocars and a camera attached to a fiber-optic scope is used so the surgeons can see what they are doing on specialized video screens.

Laparoscopy and robotic surgery are very similar techniques in terms of outcome for the patient, but they require very different skill sets of the surgeon. Some surgeons prefer one technique over the other, but both give the same result to the patient. Minimally invasive surgery allows a shorter hospital stay, usually only one night, and a faster post-operative recovery, as well as lower blood loss and fewer wound infections than open surgery. It should be noted that both laparoscopy and robotic surgery are associated with an increased rate of injury to the urinary tract over open surgery.

Many groups have reported their results on both laparoscopy and robotic laparoscopy for treatment of endometrial cancer. These results suggest that both approaches are safe and both give the same surgical result (usually as measured by numbers of lymph nodes obtained) as the traditional open surgery (called laparotomy). In general, the actual operating time is longer with minimally invasive surgery, but the length of hospital stay and amount of blood loss is much lower.

In general, the actual operating time is longer with minimally invasive surgery, but the length of hospital stay and amount of blood loss is much lower.

Obese women may benefit from the minimally invasive approach because they will not need to have a long abdominal incision. Obese women with endometrial cancer who undergo laparotomy are at high risk for wound infection and/or wound breakdown (opening of the skin) that can require lengthy wound care.

Joan said:

The referral I got from the customer I work with (an oncologist from another state) was for a doctor who performed robotic surgery. When I met with that surgeon, I was not a candidate for robotics but we did decide on total laparoscopic surgery. It made a tremendous difference to my recuperation and time off work.

37. What happens after surgery? My doctor mentioned radiation treatment but I don't get what that means.

The need for more treatment is determined by the stage of the cancer. This stage can only be determined by looking at the uterus and lymph nodes under the microscope. **Radiation** is a treatment that is given to a particular part of the body in order to kill cancer cells. These cells can be microscopic cells; in this case, radiation is used as an "extra" treatment to prevent recurrence. Radiation can also be used to treat recurrent disease if it is localized to one area of the body. It is given by a specialized physician known as a radiation oncologist.

There are different kinds of radiation. Radiation is most commonly given via a machine called a linear accelerator. These are large machines that look a little like a CAT scan machine. There is a bed for the patient to lie on and the radiation is delivered from the machine to the patient. Radiation can be given externally to treat the entire pelvic area (called whole pelvic radiation) and can also be given as an implant. An example of this is vaginal radiation, also called vaginal **brachytherapy**. In this case iridium is often used to localize the radiation to the top of the vagina.

When you first go to the radiation oncologist, the doctor will take a thorough history of your health and the treatment to date for your cancer. He or she will review your pathology and any x-rays that you may have had. The radiation oncologist will also perform a physical examination. In the case of endometrial cancer, the radiation oncologist will be checking to be sure you have completely healed from your hysterectomy. This examination will also include a pelvic examination to

Radiation

Treatment that is given to a particular part of the body in order to kill cancer cells.

Brachytherapy

A method of radiation treatment in which the source of radiation is placed close to the surface of the body or within a body cavity (Example: vagina).

37

be sure that the top of your vagina, called the vaginal "cuff," has completely healed.

Your doctor may recommend an aggressive radiation treatment plan if he or she believes you to be at risk for recurrence in the pelvis. Factors such as the tumor grade (grade 2 or 3) and deep involvement of the myometrium may play into this perceived increased risk. If recommended, it is called whole pelvic radiation. After your examination, your radiation oncologist will schedule you for a "simulation." This means that the radiation team will obtain x-rays of you, usually a CT scan of your pelvis, to assess the area of treatment (called a "field"). They will also be looking to see where normal structures, such as bowel and bladder, are located. This will allow them to map out your radiation treatment to maximize the dose to the area to be treated while minimizing the dose to the normal bowel and bladder, which are also in the pelvis. There are physicists in the radiation oncology department who help to plan the radiation fields.

Field

The area of treatment.

Some radiation oncologists will put tattoos on your body to mark out the areas to be radiated. These tattoos are very small blue dots that are not noticeable but will allow the technician to position you in the correct position under the radiation machine every time you come in to be treated.

Whole pelvic radiation is usually started between 4–8 weeks after your surgery, though it is sometimes delayed for a variety of reasons.

Whole pelvic radiation is usually started between 4–8 weeks after your surgery, though it is sometimes delayed for a variety of reasons. Once it is started, it is important to finish the treatment without delays if possible. The treatment is given daily for 5–6 weeks, but not on the weekends. Each treatment takes a very short time (less than 30 minutes). You can expect to come to radiation oncology, check in, and then wait for your appointment. You undress, put on a gown, and are positioned on the machine. The treatment is given; then you dress and go home. The entire visit should not take more than two hours each day.

While you are being treated with whole pelvic radiation therapy, you may experience some side effects. These usually do not start until 10–14 days into your treatment and may include diarrhea and fatigue. Most of the side effects can be managed with over-the-counter medications. Long-term side effects of radiation include problems with your bowel and bladder and swelling in your legs. Fortunately these side effects are infrequent.

Another form of radiation is delivered to the vagina, and is called vaginal brachytherapy. Your radiation oncologist will check to make sure that the top of the vagina is completely healed and that there is no evidence of early disease recurrence. Then he or she will fit you with a vaginal "cylinder," which is a thin metal tube like a tampon that fits into the vagina. The vaginal treatments are given with an isotope called iridium in most cases. Usually, three treatments are given. Each treatment takes 10 minutes and the treatments can be given weekly.

Your doctor may recommend that you have vaginal brachytherapy only. The treatment is intended to decrease the risk of endometrial cancer coming back at the top of the vagina, which is one of the most common places for endometrial cancer to recur. In addition, your doctor may recommend this treatment if you have invasion of your cancer into the muscle of the uterus. One of the

Treatment of Epithelial Cancers of the Uterus

most important side effects is vaginal stenosis, or closure. This can be avoided if you are sexually active or if you use a vaginal dilator at least once per week. For others, your doctor may recommend that you have both vaginal brachytherapy and whole pelvic radiation. In this case, you may have the vaginal brachytherapy done before or during the whole pelvic radiation treatment.

Intensity modulated radiation therapy (IMRT)

A form of external radiation that allows for precise planning of radiation treatment, with an aim to spare normal tissue as much as possible.

An alternative to traditional whole pelvic or vaginal radiation is called **intensity modulated radiation therapy (IMRT)**. This is a form of external radiation, but allows for precise planning of radiation treatment, with an aim to spare normal tissue as much as possible. Each treatment is delivered in multiple segments, which maximizes the treatment dose to the area of the tumor and then minimizes the radiation dose as treatment fields approach normal tissue. By varying the intensity of each dose of radiation, it can allow for the maximal treatment effect at the least risk to non-cancerous tissue.

Your radiation oncologist will likely continue to follow you after your treatment is completed. He or she will want to know about any problems you may be having with your bladder or bowel. Rarely, women can have radiation-related bowel problems, especially rectal bleeding, also called radiation proctitis. Also rare are radiation bladder problems, called radiation cystitis. These problems can be diagnosed and treated with proctoscopy in the case of the rectum or cystoscopy for the bladder. Women who have had pelvic lymph node dissections and then had whole pelvic radiation are at higher risk for having swelling in their lower extremities. This can be treated with pressure stockings and by keeping the legs elevated when possible. In extreme cases lymphedema pumps and physical therapy can be used.

Beyond radiation, your doctor may recommend chemotherapy, particularly if you have positive lymph nodes, or if you have uterine serous papillary carcinoma. The optimal treatment for endometrial cancer following surgery is not known and many **clinical trials** are being done to answer important questions about the value of radiation and chemotherapy and to understand how to combine them. You may consider being treated on one of these clinical trials. One good place to get information about clinical trials you might be eligible for is the NCI's website www.clinicaltrials.gov.

Clinical trial

A study of a new treatment, following rigorous guidelines and principles that govern clinical research in people, which are designed to ensure the scientific merit of the study, patient safety, and patient independence.

Joan said:

I really recommend second opinions for additional treatment decisions. There are so many different approaches plus possible clinical trials available. It is a huge decision and the final say is your own. At the very least, become friends with the leading cancer center websites and also the American Cancer Society and National Cancer Institute sites. Read everything you can find. No one will look out for your well-being as conscientiously as you.

38. What is the role of radiation treatment for uterine cancer?

Radiation therapy treats a particular part of the body and not the whole body. Endometrial cancer, if it recurs, is most likely to come back at the top of the vagina. In high-risk cases, recurrence is 50% local (in the pelvis) and 50% systemic (anywhere in the body). Pelvic radiation is used to decrease the risk of local recurrence (pelvis and vagina). Women who have a cancer that is deeply invasive into the muscle or high grade cancer may consider radiation therapy to decrease the risk of local recurrence.

39. How do you decide if I need radiation therapy?

The decision to treat with radiation therapy is made on the basis of risk factors found at the time of surgery.

As we mention in Question 40, the decision to treat with radiation therapy is made on the basis of risk factors found at the time of surgery. These include the grade of the tumor, the depth of invasion into the uterine muscle, the presence of tumor in vascular spaces within the muscle, the presence of tumor in the cervix, and the status of the lymph nodes if removed. Women with tumor that is considered "high risk" should have post-operative radiation.

Women with "intermediate risk" tumors may or may not benefit from radiation treatment and should discuss treatment with their doctors. They may decide to be treated only with vaginal radiation. Table 2 gives criteria of what defines risk in endometrial adenocarcinoma.

Table 2   Risk Groups and Endometrial Cancer

Risk group	
Low	Stage I Grade 1-2
Intermediate	Stage I Grade 3 Stage II Grade 1-2 Alternatively: deeply invasive OR lymphovascular invasion OR Grade 2-3: Age 70 or over: 1/3 present Age 50–69: 2/3 present Age <50: 3/3 present
High	Stage II Grade 3 Uterine Papillary serous cancers Clear cell cancers Stage III-IV

Joan said:

I read about and asked about IMRT radiation therapy There are fewer side effects—well, at least they tend to be less severe. I talked with both of the radiology oncologists I met with about this type of radiation therapy. I didn't want to demand the treatment if it did not meet the needs of my diagnosis. This is where trusting your doctors comes in—working as a team for your best care. It was agreed that this therapy would work well and it would cause less severe side effects and possibly cause less long-term problems.

40. If I don't have my uterus, what exactly is being radiated?

Vaginal treatment is directed to the top of the vagina. Cells from the uterine cancer can potentially stick here and grow at the top of the vagina, called the "vaginal cuff." This growth may be prevented by treatment of the vaginal cuff with radiation.

Whole pelvic radiation therapy treats the pelvis—the area where the pelvic nodes are and also where the tissue next to the uterus is. This treatment will prevent recurrence in these areas. Sometimes the radiation doctor may also elect to treat the lymph nodes along the aorta and vena cava, called the para-aortic lymph nodes.

Joan said:

This is a big puzzle and the question everyone in my family asked too. Isn't it empty space now? It seemed weird that with everything taken out during surgery there was anything left to address. I'm sure this question is asked of every oncologist by every patient. It isn't a "hole" but filled with cells and tissue that you need to keep healthy.

41. Will I need chemotherapy?

If you have positive lymph nodes or if you have involvement of the ovaries or tubes, you will likely need chemotherapy. In addition, if you have a serous papillary cancer of the uterus, your doctor will almost certainly recommend chemotherapy regardless of the stage of your disease. Finally, for disease that has reached the bowel or bladder, involves the upper abdomen or beyond (Stage III or IV), the standard of care is to offer chemotherapy.

In most cases, chemotherapy is not being given to treat cancer that was left behind, because most of the time your surgeon believes he or she has removed all of the cancer. Sometimes there can be cancer cells "floating" in your body, either in your abdomen (also called the peritoneal cavity) or in your circulation. The chemotherapy is being given to kill these cells so that they don't have a chance to stop floating and sit and grow somewhere in your body.

In most cases, chemotherapy is not being given to treat cancer that was left behind, because most of the time your surgeon believes he or she has removed all of the cancer.

42. What kind of chemotherapy is used to treat uterine cancer?

Platinum salts
Drugs that commonly serve as the basis for treatment of endometrial cancer.

Drugs known as **platinum salts** serve as the basis for treatment of endometrial cancer. The current data supports a three-drug combination of cisplatin, doxorubicin, and paclitaxel. However, it is quite a difficult treatment to tolerate. Therefore, another combination is frequently given, which employs carboplatin and paclitaxel. The optimal chemotherapy treatment for endometrial cancer is still being studied and you may choose to enter a clinical trial for treatment.

Cisplatin works by breaking up the DNA of cells, causing them to undergo cell death, or apoptosis. It is given by vein (intravenously, or IV). It is a powerful drug that, unfortunately, also affects normal cells, which is responsible for its side effects. Common side effects include severe nausea and vomiting, kidney problems, numbness and tingling, and ringing in the ears. Fortunately, there are good drugs to help prevent or even treat the nausea and vomiting. The other side effects tend to happen as treatment continues, and your doctor will ask if any are present. If they are, he or she might have to decrease the dose or even stop this drug so the symptoms do not become worse.

Fortunately, another drug of the same class as cisplatin is available. It is called carboplatin and, unlike cisplatin, it is not as toxic to normal cells and its side effects are in turn different. It causes problems with blood counts, particularly platelets, which can put you at risk for bleeding complications. It can also cause nausea and vomiting, but not to the same degree as cisplatin.

Doxorubicin works by interfering with the DNA as well. It is usually given as a slow IV push in the chemotherapy unit and it is critical that the IV is working as it should because if it leaks out of the vein and into your soft tissue, it can cause a very severe chemical burn. Doxorubicin also causes problems with blood counts, nausea, and vomiting. Its most serious complication though affects your heart. If you get too much of it (over your lifetime), then it can make the heart weak, a condition called a **cardiomyopathy**. Fortunately, oncologists have worked out the safe dosing of doxorubicin so as to stay clear of this risk. If your doctor decides that you need more than the accepted risk allows, there is a drug available to protect your heart from doxorubicin caused damage. This drug is called dexrazoxane.

Cardiomyopathy

Weakening of the heart muscle causing it not to function well.

45

Paclitaxel works by stopping cancer cells as they divide, which causes them to die. It is also an IV drug and is delivered over a 3-hour time period in most cases. Its major toxicities are hair loss (which happens after the very first treatment), numbness and tingling, and joint aches and pains. It can also cause an allergic-type reaction when it is first given. Symptoms can include flushing of the skin, a sensation of heat, coughing, rapid heartbeat, high blood pressure, and chest tightness. In order to prevent this, you will need to take steroids before the treatment. If the first dose goes well with premedication, then you may not need to take steroids again, but this should be discussed with your doctor.

Your doctor may talk to you about being treated with progesterone therapy. This is not a chemotherapy agent, but is a hormone that is sometimes used if a woman has something called a positive "washing." Your surgeon will pour sterile fluid into your abdomen and suction this off right before your hysterectomy. If cells are found in this fluid but your cancer is otherwise low risk for recurrence (low grade, minimal muscle invasion, negative lymph nodes), your doctor may talk to you about taking progesterone. The most common progesterone used in this case is called megestrol acetate.

Joan said:

Each oncologist has their own approach to treatment (this is true for radiation also). Sometimes it depends on what trials they are involved in or what papers they are writing. Along with most modern medicine, cancer treatments and medications are changing all the time. You just have to be comfortable that your doctor is at the forefront of the information and trust that the approach the doctor recommends is the proper one for your type/level of cancer and for you.

43. How is chemotherapy given?

As previously discussed, all of the chemotherapy for endometrial cancer is given by vein. One of the drugs, doxorubicin, can be particularly dangerous if it leaks out of an intravenous drip (IV) into the skin. In that case, it can cause a chemical burn, which can become very serious if untreated. For this reason, women with poor venous access or who are not good with needles sometimes opt for a **mediport** (see Question 47). These will allow for easier infusion access. While it is more convenient, they are not absolutely required for everyone getting chemotherapy.

Mediport

A temporary device that is surgically implanted in the chest or arm to accept an IV during chemotherapy.

Joan said:

I have it intravenously. It takes about 6-7 hours for the whole treatment. The steroids you are given make you feel energized the next day but they also kept me from sleeping! Not a good trade-off in that I'm working fulltime. The first time I went, a friend took me which helped pass the time. There are 3-4 pre-medications given and then the cancer drugs (I get carbo/paclitaxel). The facility I go to has two reclining chairs per room so it isn't like some production line of sick people!

The nursing staff—these front line people—are a good resource also for getting a handle on the specific side effects your medications may cause.

44. What are the side effects of treatment?

We touched on this briefly before, but in general, chemotherapy can cause lowering of the blood cell counts, which may put you at an increased risk for infection, anemia, or bleeding, hair loss, nausea, diarrhea, membrane irritation, and may induce premature menopause, which can present as hot flashes and vaginal dryness or

Loss of hair on the head, eyebrows, eyelashes, and genitals is distressing and affects a female's perception of her sexual attractiveness.

atrophy. Loss of hair on the head, eyebrows, eyelashes, and genitals is distressing and affects a female's perception of her sexual attractiveness. Chemotherapy-induced early ovarian failure causes menopausal symptoms like hot flashes, sleep problems, vaginal dryness, and mood problems. Vaginal dryness can become a serious medical concern and often leads to painful intercourse on penetration. However, each drug that is used in endometrial cancer can cause specific side effects.

Cisplatin can cause profound nausea and vomiting, which may persist as much as 7–10 days out from treatment. It can also cause the kidneys to malfunction and a permanent numbness and tingling (or neuropathy). Carboplatin, its cousin, is a lot kinder to patients. It can cause some nausea, but its major toxicity is to lower platelets (which can make you prone to bleeding).

Dyspnea on exertion

Shortness of breath during activities like walking, sometimes a side effect of chemotherapy in which the heart muscle is weakened.

Doxorubicin can affect your heart muscle if a threshold is surpassed. This can present as shortness of breath during activities like walking (called **dyspnea on exertion**) or even difficulty breathing during sleep. This is due to the weakening of the heart muscle, which can cause congestive heart failure. For this reason, your doctor will pay close attention to the doses you are receiving and may order a baseline heart scan prior to the start of treatment to get a good look at how well your heart is working.

Paclitaxel can affect nerves and can cause numbness or tingling, usually noted in the hands and feet. Patients may also run the risk of developing an allergic reaction when it is given. To prevent this, you may be told to take steroids prior to treatment.

Joan said:

The first three to six days were my worst. The muscle aches and joint pain were tough. I am not one to take more medication than the label says or what is suggested. I probably should have called the chemo unit nurse but it fell on the weekend and I would have had to talk to the doctor on call. I figured weathering it was what it was all about. WRONG. When I went for my next session, I asked the chemo nurse about upping my pain reliever and she said there was no problem with doubling it for that short time frame. Oh, I should have called that first time!!

Overall, a loss of mental acuity ("cancer brain") has become a fact of life for now. I frequently have to search for the right word. Fatigue is becoming more pronounced as I progress through my treatment sessions. I am still working full time but look forward to lying down after work for a much needed rest. I don't often sleep but the resting helps. I also found my face to be extremely itchy. I didn't lose my eyebrows but as they and my lashes and facial hair thinned out, the dying follicles made my face itch.

I did lose most of my hair the second week after my first chemo session (the time frame is different for each drug given, so ask). I had bought a wig and had shaved off my hair the week before it started falling out. I had already noticed more than normal hair amounts on the comb in the mornings. I didn't want to have gobs of hair in my hands some morning when I was washing my hair. My scalp was painful a couple of days before—it's true that your hair can hurt. I find I'm more comfortable in scarves and turbans than in my wig. Although when I work with customers, I know me being in a wig is more comfortable for them.

45. My doctor says I have advanced cancer of the uterus. Can I still be cured?

Cancer that has spread beyond the uterus is not generally curable. The rate of surviving five years decreases dramatically as the stage increases. That is, women with Stage I disease have a 75%–95% chance of living five years. For Stage II, it drops to 50%; Stage III it is 30%; and for Stage IV it is less than 5%. Still, while not curable, it is treatable, and while as the cancer advances cure is not possible, a remission or getting the cancer to stop growing would be reasonable options. There are many approaches to treat endometrial cancer, and with the research underway, hopefully these options will continue to expand.

There are many approaches to treat endometrial cancer, and with the research underway, hopefully these options will continue to expand.

Joan said:

I chose not to read about the survival rate of my type/grade of cancer—I avoided that specific statistic. I didn't want a "dying" number in my head ricocheting around. I did learn about each treatment's extension of survivability—it was part of the decision making process. It wasn't until I read this manuscript that I learned what the survival average is for me. Now I am faced with not letting myself dwell on it. I view my case as individually as I can and know that I will conquer this and live a long and wonderful life.

46. How will my age affect my options for treatment?

We do not, in general, make treatment decisions based on age. What is more important is how you are physically doing when you are diagnosed; a 45-year-old woman with end-stage complications from diabetes may be less able to handle chemotherapy than a 70-year-old woman in good health. That is, your ability to perform your own activities of daily living and take care of your own needs (sometimes called a performance status) can tell your doctor more than merely focusing attention to your age. The various treatments, from surgery to radiation to chemotherapy, all have risks and a balanced consideration of the benefits and the risks of treatment are always required.

Joan said:

At 58, I am still young in that I have/want another 30 years ahead of me. I want aggressive treatment balanced with minimal long-term side effects. It takes asking question after question of your doctors to learn ALL you can. This is a case of knowing what questions to ask. There is nothing you can't ask your doctors!

47. What is a mediport? Should I get one?

As we mentioned in Question 43, a mediport is a means of giving chemotherapy. As opposed to an intravenous catheter, which is placed and then removed after it is done, a mediport is called a central access device. It is surgically placed underneath the skin and is designed for long-term use. Because it is under the skin and no part of it is sticking out from the skin, the risk of an infection is very low. The part you can feel is called the reservoir and the surface of this part (called the septum) is where a needle is inserted. The reservoir is attached via tubing that sits in one of the large veins of your arm, neck, or chest. In addition to chemotherapy, it can be used to infuse intravenous fluids, nutrition, antibiotics, and any other medication that must be given directly into the bloodstream. The indications for a mediport are essentially centered on the person receiving chemotherapy: the duration of treatment, the state of her own veins in the arms (which will determine if they can be accessed), and patient's own requests, all fall into the decision on whether or not a port should be placed.

PART FIVE

Uterine Sarcomas

Are there different types of uterine sarcoma?

What kind of treatment is given for sarcomas?

What is my prognosis?

More . . .

48. What is a sarcoma?

As we briefly touched on in Question 9, the uterus can give rise to different kinds of tumors. Those that develop out of the muscle or supporting tissue of the uterus are called **sarcomas**. These are very different from the endometrial cancers discussed earlier, both in their behavior and their prognosis.

49. Are there different types of uterine sarcoma?

There are three main types of sarcomas of the uterus. Those that arise from the muscle are called leiomyosarcomas and account for about 30% of all sarcomas of the uterus. They can occur at any age but the majority occur in women in their fifties. A more common type typically seen in postmenopausal women, and that accounts for up to 50% of these cancers, are **carcinosarcomas**. These are dual cancers with an epithelial component (carcino-) and the sarcoma component. They can also arise in the ovary and other sites in the female tract but are commonly seen in the uterus. In carcinosarcomas, the muscular-cancer can appear as tissue that is native to the uterus (called homologous) or interestingly, it can grow as tissue that is not normally found in the uterus, such as bone or cartilage (called heterologous). Finally, there are **endometrial stromal sarcomas**, which do not arise from the muscle, but from the supporting tissue of the uterus (called the **stroma**). These account for about 15% of tumors and typically are responsive to estrogen. There are other rare sarcomas, such as adenosarcomas, which unlike carcinosarcomas have a non-malignant epithelial component (the "adeno-" part), and rhabdomyosarcomas, but the most common ones are those previously listed.

Sarcoma

Tumor that develops out of the muscle or supporting tissue of the uterus.

Carcinosarcomas

Dual cancers with an epithelial component (carcino-) and the sarcoma component.

Endometrial stromal sarcomas

Cancers which do not arise from the muscle, but from the supporting tissue of the uterus (called the stroma).

Stroma

Supporting tissue of the uterus.

50. Are there risk factors for uterine sarcomas?

The only established risk factor is prior pelvic radiation, which is associated with 10% to 25% of these types of cancers. There is a very small risk of uterine sarcomas, particularly for carcinosarcomas, in women who take Tamoxifen. Otherwise, there are no other known risk factors for this.

51. Are there symptoms for uterine sarcomas?

There are no specific symptoms for uterine sarcomas. The signs of a potential uterine cancer apply to these tumors as well. Thus, any evidence of abnormal bleeding (i.e., not part of a normal menses, postmenopausal bleeding, or particularly heavy bleeding), a sensation of abdominal pain or fullness, increased frequency of urination, or a mass in the vagina, are all signs of uterine cancer, and may be seen with uterine sarcomas.

There are no specific symptoms for uterine sarcomas.

52. What kind of surgery is done for uterine sarcomas?

Both the diagnosis and staging of uterine sarcomas have been adapted by the approach to endometrial cancers. Surgery is still the mainstay of treatment and the approach is determined by how large and/or how advanced the cancer is at diagnosis. The lymph nodes are at risk for being involved with carcinosarcomas, so a node dissection is performed. However, a study from Memorial Sloan-Kettering Cancer Center suggests that if leiomyosarcomas are isolated to the uterus or pelvis, then the lymph nodes are not usually involved. Given this, women who have leiomyosarcomas should have nodes removed only if their surgeon feels they look

Uterine Sarcomas

suspicious. For any woman with uterine cancer, though, a careful inspection of the entire abdomen and pelvis is required. Surgery is best performed by a Gynecologic Oncologist.

The staging of uterine sarcomas has been separated from that of endometrial cancers in the most recent FIGO classification system. It is as follows:

For Leiomyosarcomas and Endometrial Stromal Sarcomas

Stage	Definition
I	Tumor limited to uterus
IA	Tumor size up to 5 cm
IB	Tumor size over 5 cm
II	Tumor extends to the pelvis
IIA	Ovarian involvement
IIB	Tumor extends to pelvic tissue beyond the uterus
III	Tumor invades tissue in the abdomen
IIIA	Tumor involves one site
IIIB	Tumor involves more than one site
IIIC	Metastasis to the lymph nodes of the pelvis and/or para-aortic area
IV	
IVA	Tumor invades bladder and/or rectum
IVB	Distant metastasis

For Adenosarcomas

Stage	Definition
I	Tumor limited to uterus
IA	Tumor limited to endometrium/endocervix with no myometrial invasion
IB	Tumor with less than or equal to half myometrial invasion
IC	Tumor with more than half myometrial invasion
II	Tumor extends to the pelvis
IIA	Ovarian involvement
IIB	Tumor extends to extrauterine pelvic tissue
III	Tumor invades abdominal tissues
IIIA	One site involved
IIIB	Tumor is at more than one site
IIIC	Metastasis to pelvic and/or para-aortic lymph nodes
IV	
IVA	Tumor invades bladder and/or rectum
IVB	Distant metastasis

Carcinosarcomas continue to be staged as endometrial adenocarcinomas.

53. What kind of treatment is given for sarcomas?

We have no evidence that treatment after surgery is of benefit for women with uterine sarcomas, and this applies to both the use of chemotherapy and to the use of radiation therapy. However, treatment with chemotherapy or radiation (or both) is highly individualized to the patient and her physician's preference.

Radiation can be directed to the pelvis only or may be given to the entire abdomen, and much depends on what type of sarcoma you have and how extensive it was when found.

Women with carcinosarcomas were studied in a large randomized trial where half received whole abdominal radiation and the other half a combination chemotherapy regimen using the drugs ifosfamide and cisplatin. This study showed that chemotherapy reduced the risk of recurrence by 30% and also improved survival over radiation alone. This suggests that chemotherapy may play a large role in treating these specific sarcomas.

54. What is my prognosis?

Uterine sarcomas are generally very aggressive, though the risk of having it return is most closely linked to grade and stage. That is, grade 3 sarcomas are more likely to come back than grade 1 tumors, and those that have spread beyond the uterus are more likely to return than those isolated to the uterus. Even so, women who have had leiomyosarcomas run the risk of having it return despite the stage and despite treatment after surgery. An often quoted risk is 50:50 with or without chemotherapy or radiation. Given this, a frank discussion with your doctor is very important when you are considering further treatment beyond surgery.

If your tumor recurs, then your doctor may recommend a repeat surgery to remove it. This is more likely if you have only one tumor seen or if you have recurred after a long time. If, after radiation or chemotherapy, the tumor grows quickly back, however, it is not likely that surgery will provide you any benefit. In either case, further treatment beyond surgery will be recommended. Standard drugs used for sarcomas include doxorubicin or docetaxel and gemcitabine (for leiomyosarcomas), or carboplatin and paclitaxel (for carcinosarcomas). Endometrial stromal sarcomas are treated with doxorubicin-based therapies.

PART SIX

Gestational Trophoblast Neoplasias

What is gestational trophoblast neoplasia?

How are moles treated? Will I need a hysterectomy?

Can I have children after being diagnosed with this?

More . . .

55. What is gestational trophoblast neoplasia?

Gestational trophoblastic neoplasia (GTN) constitutes a very rare group of tumors that can grow from cells inside a woman's uterus. Unlike endometrial cancer, which arises from the lining of the uterus called the endometrium, GTN arises from the cells that normally make a placenta (afterbirth) during a pregnancy. **Trophoblast** refers to the specialized cells that normally surround an embryo. These cells ultimately will make the placenta that will feed the fetus during the pregnancy. Sometimes the fertilization process is abnormal and, instead of a normal pregnancy, a **"molar pregnancy"** results from abnormal development of the trophoblast. This abnormal pregnancy can be a "complete mole" meaning that it consists of all trophoblast and no fetus, or a "partial mole" meaning that there is also fetal tissue present. This fetal tissue is always abnormal because the partial mole is "triploid"—has three sets of DNA chromosomes rather than the normal two. A complete **hydatidiform mole** most often develops when either 1 or 2 sperm cells fertilize an "empty" egg cell (a cell that contains no nucleus or DNA). All the genes come from the sperm cell. These moles are usually XX. A partial mole occurs when two sperm fertilize a normal egg. All partial moles are "triploid" for this reason: XXY or XYY.

A complete mole can metastasize (spread). The molar pregnancy can invade into the uterus and can spread to distant organs, usually liver or lungs. Even with spread, most molar pregnancies can be cured.

Beyond molar pregnancies, there are two other types of GTN. **Choriocarcinoma** is a very aggressive form that usually develops after a complete mole, but rarely can be seen after a partial mole or even a normal pregnancy. It has the propensity to metastasize early. **Placental site trophoblastic tumor (PSTT)** develops from the place

Trophoblast
Specialized cells that normally surround an embryo and ultimately make the placenta that will feed the fetus during the pregnancy.

Molar pregnancy
Pregnancy that results from abnormal development of the trophoblast.

Hydatidiform mole
The result that most often develops when either one or two sperm cells fertilize an "empty" egg cell (a cell that contains no nucleus or DNA).

Choriocarcinoma
A very aggressive form of GTN that usually develops after a complete mole, but rarely can be seen after a partial mole or even a normal pregnancy.

Placental site trophoblastic tumor (PSTT)
A tumor that develops from the place where the placenta attaches to the endometrium.

where the placenta attaches to the endometrium. The PSTT can invade into the uterus and be very difficult to treat medically. As such, it is the only GTN where a hysterectomy may be necessitated in order to effect a cure.

As noted, these are exceedingly rare events. About 1 in every 1,500–2,000 pregnancies in the United States is a molar pregnancy. The incidence is higher in Asia for unclear reasons, affecting 1 in 120 pregnancies in that area of the world. Invasive moles affect 1 in 15,000 pregnancies and choriocarcinomas affect 1 in 40,000. Complicated twin gestations (see Question 59) where a viable fetus co-exists with a mole is exceedingly rare, seen in 1 in 22,000–100,000 pregnancies.

There are risk factors associated with GTN:

- Women under 20 and over 40
- Prior history of a molar pregnancy
- Prior miscarriages
- Being A-positive or AB-positive blood type

56. How are they diagnosed?

In GTN, the blood pregnancy test, which measures human chorionic gonadotropin (or hCG) will be extremely elevated, often much higher than what would be expected normally. In addition, the hCG does not follow the normal pattern of expression one sees in pregnancy or else, in the woman who has delivered a baby or had loss of the pregnancy, it fails to return to normal.

Beyond that, women with a complete mole may have the following signs and symptoms during the first trimester of pregnancy:

- Vaginal bleeding
- Ovarian cysts
- Uterine size that is larger than expected based on last menstrual period

- Severe nausea and vomiting
- High blood pressure very early in pregnancy
- Signs of hyperthyroidism

Similar symptoms may be seen with the other forms of GTN as well. Partial moles usually present with abnormal bleeding in the context of a pregnancy. In such cases, it would be important to rule out a miscarriage. Women with choriocarcinomas may present either as part of a missed abortion picture or after delivery of an abnormal or normal pregnancy.

It is important to note that, while the hCG is an indicator of GTN, it can also be falsely elevated. That is, the hCG test can be abnormal and you be not pregnant or have a mole. This situation is referred to as a "phantom hCG". This can happen because your body may have proteins that are interfering with the way the lab tests for hCG, usually because proteins are reacting to the test. If the hCG is the only evidence of a problem, it must be repeated. Your doctor can even test for it in your urine. In phantom hCG, the level is usually normal. In addition, there are special reference laboratories that can check your blood for any factors that may cause this abnormal report. The importance of recognizing phantom hCG is that women have been misdiagnosed with GTN and gone through chemotherapy inappropriately. Knowing whether the hCG is a real result or is false will hopefully prevent women from being exposed to chemotherapy that is not needed.

The importance of recognizing phantom hCG is that women have been misdiagnosed with GTN and gone through chemotherapy inappropriately.

57. Is imaging helpful in making this diagnosis?

Ultrasound is very sensitive and reliable for diagnosing both complete and partial moles. An ultrasound will reveal a "snowstorm" pattern inside the uterus and, in cases of a complete mole, there will be no evidence of a fetal heartbeat or fetal parts. There may also be evidence of many ovarian cysts, which can be associated with complete mole. The presence of a fetus supports the diagnosis of a partial mole.

Women with PSTT may have an abnormal lesion identified by ultrasound. Alternatively, it may appear to be an area of abnormal signaling on ultrasound, called **echogenic foci,** surrounded by areas consistent with blood, called hemorrhagic cysts. If taken in the context of a pregnancy or as new onset bleeding in a woman who has already delivered her baby, this diagnosis should be ruled out.

Echogenic foci

An area of abnormal signaling on ultrasound.

58. How are moles treated? Will I need a hysterectomy?

Both complete and partial moles are treated with a D&C to empty the uterus. Prior to the procedure, your doctor will check a chest x-ray to make sure that there is no evidence of disease in the chest. Your doctor will also check to make sure your thyroid function is normal, that your blood chemistry is normal, and that you are not significantly anemic as these factors may complicate your procedure.

The cervix is dilated (opened) and the contents of the uterus are completely removed. Looking at the tissue under the microscope makes the diagnosis of a complete or partial mole. It is important to stress that there is usually no viable fetus present in either of these diagnoses.

In most cases a hysterectomy is not required. After the procedure, the doctor will check blood tests to make sure the pregnancy blood test numbers come back to normal.

Only in the case of PSTT, which is very rare, may a hysterectomy be needed.

Only in the case of PSTT, which is very rare, may a hysterectomy be needed.

59. How does this diagnosis impact a pregnant woman? Will my baby survive?

In complete moles, there is no baby present; in partial moles, the fetus is usually malformed or appears inappropriate for the expected age, or is usually not present at all, though fetal parts can be identified on ultrasound. In both cases, the fetus is not expected to go to term, let alone survive, and all cases end in a spontaneous abortion or miscarriage.

In extremely rare circumstances, a normal pregnancy may coexist with a mole. This situation is referred to as a "twin pregnancy." There are fewer than 200 cases reported in the medical literature, and most are associated with the use of technology to have a baby, or assisted reproductive technologies. Twin pregnancies are a high-risk situation, and all cases should be referred to specialists in high-risk pregnancies (maternal fetal medicine) and to gynecologic oncologists. There is hope that your baby can survive even with a coexisting mole, but it is a very serious situation that requires input from specialists.

60. Can I have children after being diagnosed with this?

Most women diagnosed with a partial or complete mole will have a complete recovery with only a D&C.

Most women diagnosed with a partial or complete mole will have a complete recovery with only a D&C. These women will almost certainly be able to conceive a normal pregnancy following the diagnosis; however, they are at increased risk over the general population to have a second molar pregnancy. Therefore, it is recommended that women get an early ultrasound with subsequent pregnancies to exclude a recurrent mole. Still, pregnancy is possible after the diagnosis of GTN; even after choriocarcinoma treatment, patients can still have normal pregnancies. For women with PSTT, if a hysterectomy has been done, then you will not be able to carry your own child; if the ovaries were spared, however, you could still undergo in vitro fertilization to create embryos, who can then be transferred to another woman (called a gestational surrogate) to carry for you. For more on fertility and pregnancy, see Questions 83 and 84.

61. How curable is this?

GTN is very curable. Partial and complete moles can be cured with surgery alone (D&C). If the hCG blood test remains elevated or rises, or if there is evidence of metastasis, chemotherapy is given. Chemotherapy is highly curative in this disease, even when there are metastases to the liver or lungs.

Partial and complete moles can be cured with surgery alone (D&C).

62. How is it staged?

There are two different staging systems for GTN. One is released by the International Federation of Obstetrics and Gynecology (FIGO). It describes the extent of disease spread (Table 3). Notably, disease that has spread to lungs is considered as Stage III, whereas disease involving any other organ (like the liver or brain) is considered Stage IV. This reflects the different risks a woman faces with GTN and the fact that spread to the lungs is not as serious as having it go to other organs.

The other system is called the modified **World Health Organization (WHO) scoring system** (Table 4). This system is used for women with persistent or metastatic disease to assist in choosing appropriate treatment.

World Health Organization (WHO) scoring system

System used to assist in choosing appropriate treatment for women with persistent or metastatic disease.

The "score" is calculated based on certain prognostic factors for having persistent disease. These include your age, whether a pregnancy was associated with it (and if so, the time that elapsed from the pregnancy to the diagnosis), areas of disease, and whether or not prior treatment was given. The important thing to know is that the score can change if the disease comes back. That is, even if you started out with one score, your doctor will re-do the scoring system if you relapse.

Table 3   The FIGO Staging System for Gestational Trophoblast Neoplasia

Stage I	Confined to the uterus
Stage II	Outside the uterus, in the vagina, ovaries or tissue next to the uterus
Stage III	Extends to lungs
Stage IV	All other sites

Table 4   WHO Scoring System for GTN

Scores	0	1	3	4
Age	<40	≥40	–	–
Previous pregnancy	Mole	Abortion	Term	–
Months since pregnancy	<4	4–<7	7–<13	≥13
hCG value	<1000	1000–<10,000	10^4–<10^5	>10^5
Largest tumor size	–	3–<5 cm	>5 cm	
Sites of metastases	Lung	Spleen, kidney	GI	Liver, brain
Number of metastases		1–4	5–8	>8
Previously used chemotherapy			Single drug	2 or more drugs

63. How is it treated?

Molar pregnancies are treated with D&C. The level of blood pregnancy test is then followed weekly until it is non-detectable. Sometimes there is persistent disease; this is diagnosed by a continued elevated blood pregnancy test. If that happens, it is assumed that there are still abnormal trophoblastic cells present. These can be treated with single agent therapy and either methotrexate or actinomycin-D is used. If you have choriocarcinoma, or if your WHO score is 7 or over, then you face a higher risk of relapsed disease. In this case, more complicated regimens are used, such as etoposide, methotrexate and actinomycin-D (EMA) alternating with cyclophosphamide and vincristine (CO), also known as EMA-CO. For PSTT or persistent GTN despite EMA-CO, a variation is used where the EMA alternates with etoposide and cisplatin, known as EMA-EP. If you require chemotherapy beyond single agents, it is best to be seen by someone who is an expert in the management of GTN.

Etoposide is given by IV and works by blocking the function of the protein, topoisomerase, which is involved in stabilizing DNA. Its side effects are hair loss, diarrhea or constipation, a metallic taste that can develop, and lowering of blood counts. It also carries a risk of injury to the bone marrow and can cause leukemia later on in life.

Methotrexate blocks the folate pathway, an important vitamin pathway in the body that is involved in the creation of DNA and RNA. It too can affect the bone marrow, but may also have a negative effect on the gastrointestinal system. Patients receiving methotrexate can develop sores or ulcers all along their GI system from their mouth down the esophagus, and even involving the colon and rectum. It can also lead to liver inflammation and cause lung injury which, in the latter, may present as a dry cough.

Actinomycin-D is an anticancer antibiotic, and works by blocking the synthesis of DNA. It, too, will cause general chemotherapy side effects including fatigue, lowering of blood counts, hair loss, and mouth sores.

Cyclophosphamide is a very old drug, available as an IV and oral (PO) formulation. For GTN, it is given IV. It is actually a **pro-drug**, which means it is converted to an anticancer drug after it enters the body. This conversion occurs in your liver. It causes the usual side effects of treatment, including nausea, vomiting, lowering of blood counts, hair thinning, and diarrhea. It can also be toxic to the bladder and may even result in bladder cancer as a future risk, but with proper fluid given during and after treatment, this risk can be minimized.

Pro-drug

A drug which is converted by the patient's liver into an anti-cancer drug after it enters the body.

Vincristine works on dividing cells to lead them to death. It works similarly to paclitaxel and, like paclitaxel, it can cause numbness and tingling to develop. At its worst, it can cause a foot drop, which happens when you cannot turn the ankle and toes upward. You might complain that you have started to trip on your own feet as the first sign of this. Vincristine can also cause significant constipation due to its effects on the nervous system of the gut. It is important to watch for these symptoms and to let your doctor know about them before they get serious.

Your hCG will be followed every 10–14 days on treatment, and as long as it remains elevated you will require treatment. Once it normalizes 1-2 extra cycles are given, mostly as extra insurance. Once in remission, you will need to have this level checked regularly over the next two years. You should also avoid pregnancy during this period of active follow-up. As long as the hCG is normal you should not require any further testing. However, if it starts a sustained rise (repeated twice with confirmed rises) you will need to be re-staged.

After treatment (especially with multi-agent chemotherapy) you will need to be followed for a long time, even if it is no longer with your oncologist. This is because there is a risk of a secondary cancer related to treatment, and the type of cancer risk changes the longer you are followed:

- There is a risk for leukemia up to 4 years after treatment.
- There is a risk for colon cancer between 5 and 9 years of follow-up.
- There is a risk for melanoma 10 to 14 years later.
- There is a risk for breast cancer 25 years after treatment.

Knowing these risks will be an important point to remember as you embark on follow-up as a cancer survivor.

64. What happens if GTN does not go in to remission or returns?

The risk of recurrence or progression has been associated with several factors:

- Liver involvement
- Brain involvement
- Detection of disease six months or longer from the prior pregnancy
- Term delivery

While it does not change the treatments you will receive, it is knowledge that will explain the surveillance you will need following treatment. Still, even women who have recurrent disease or disease that spreads can still be cured because GTN is very sensitive to chemotherapy. Metastatic disease is almost always curable with single drug chemotherapy. High WHO score choriocarcinoma and invasive moles that have already seen one or two lines of treatment are harder to treat and require more complicated regimens. If the tumor comes back even after multiple trials, surgery may be considered in an attempt for cure. However, women do still die of this disease and if, after multiple treatments, the cancer comes back, a frank discussion on the benefits of further treatment will be required. Fortunately, this is rarely the case, but if it happens to you, seeking out a specialist who has seen lots of these cases should be strongly considered.

Metastatic disease is almost always curable with single drug chemotherapy.

PART SEVEN

Treating Recurrent Uterine Cancer

Is surgery an option if my disease comes back?

How is uterine cancer treated once it has come back?

What is a clinical trial?

More . . .

65. How can endometrial cancer come back if I don't have my uterus?

It can be very confusing to hear your doctor say that uterine cancer has recurred. Unfortunately, uterine cancer does recur and spread, which is why women still die from it. Cancer can affect the entire body, and uterine cancer is not an exception to that. For some women, cancer cells are present outside of the uterus, and these cells cannot be picked up by the best surgeon. With time, these cells may spread to other organs by the bloodstream or lymphatic system, may implant and grow on the new surgical scar, the top of the vagina (called the vaginal cuff), or implant in the abdomen.

Cancer that has spread, or metastasized, is still attributed to the primary organ where the cancer first originated.

Cells that are in the vascular system can grow anywhere in the body, but most often they land in the lungs, and can be picked up as lung tumors. Just because they are in the lung does not mean the same thing as having lung cancer though. Cancer that has spread, or metastasized, is still attributed to the primary organ where the cancer first originated. So, in this case, it would be considered uterine cancer, metastatic to the lungs. In cases not too uncommon, lung metastases may look like primary lung cancer to the radiologist, especially if you have risk factors for lung cancer (like a long smoking history). If there is any confusion as to what is happening with newly discovered lesions, and the differential includes metastatic disease, then a biopsy is usually recommended.

Lymphoma
Primary lymph cancer.

Disease in the lymphatic system usually recurs in the lymph nodes along the aorta and vena cava or in the pelvis. As previously described, disease in the lymph nodes is considered metastatic disease, and not primary lymph cancer (or **lymphoma**). Sometimes it requires a biopsy, though, to confirm it.

The way your doctor finds out whether cancer has spread is by doing an extent of disease (EOD) evaluation. For women with uterine cancer, the hallmark of the EOD exam is the pelvic exam. Radiology studies such as CT, MRI, and fluorodeoxyglucose positron emission testing (FDG-PET) may also be used.

Biopsies can be performed as a minimally invasive procedure that does not require a trip to the operating room. If it is an area that can be reached by your gynecologic oncologist (located in the vaginal cuff, for example), he or she may take a piece of it while you are in clinic using local anesthesia. If it is in the lungs or liver, the biopsy can be done using ultrasound or computed tomography (CT) to guide the biopsy. If it is in the abdomen and otherwise not very accessible by a radiologist, your doctor may talk to you about going to the operating room and, while you are under general anesthesia, doing the procedure in surgery.

66. Is surgery an option if my disease comes back?

In select patients, surgery may be a very reasonable option. If there is evidence of isolated recurrence to one spot, or the disease returned after a year or longer, your doctor may discuss with you surgical removal. However, you will also need another form of treatment, such as radiation or chemotherapy, after surgical removal. This is because the recurrence is most likely from involvement of the lymphatic or vascular system, and cells can still implant and grow unless additional therapy is used. However, while it might be technically feasible to have surgery for recurrent disease, there is no evidence that undergoing a second surgery will improve your chances of survival. A frank discussion with your gynecologic oncologist is required before embarking on repeat surgery.

67. How is uterine cancer treated once it has come back?

Both radiation and medical therapy are used. Radiation is usually given for recurrent disease in the pelvis (sometimes referred to as a local recurrence). This is because when cancer recurs in the pelvis, it can lead to bleeding or pain and a treatment that works quickly is often desired. Radiation therapy can provide excellent symptom control, or palliation, for this kind of recurrence; however, it is not considered curative. For all other circumstances, medical therapy is used.

If the cancer is a low-grade tumor and you are not having symptoms, a conservative approach would be to try pills aimed at blocking estrogen exposure, such as Tamoxifen, or other progestin-like agents, such as Megestrol. These can help shrink down tumors, but appear to be most active in grade 1 or 2 endometrial cancers. This can also be an effective strategy in treating endometrial stromal sarcomas, which usually feed off of estrogen.

If there is a large volume of metastatic disease (involving multiple organs, for example), you are symptomatic of the cancer, high grade or worrisome histology (like serous or leiomyosarcoma) then chemotherapy is going to be recommended. For adenocarcinomas, the choices will depend on whether or not chemotherapy had already been given. If you have not received chemotherapy, then a platinum-based regimen as we discussed in detail in Question 42 would be recommended. However, if you have already seen chemotherapy, the options are fairly limited because there are no drugs approved for use in the United States in the second-line setting. Your doctor may extrapolate your treatment to how we approach other aggressive gynecologic cancers, such as ovarian cancer. In this setting, however, exploring your options for clinical trials makes sense.

In addition to paclitaxel and doxorubicin (discussed in Question 42) other standard drugs that could be used in the second-line treatment of endometrial adenocarcinoma include:

- Gemcitabine: acts to stop DNA synthesis and, by doing so, cause cell death. It primarily affects the blood counts, though women can also run a temperature 24 hours after it is given. Rarely, it can cause problems with your lungs.
- Ifosfamide: a cousin of cyclophosphamide (discussed in Question 70), it works by causing damage to DNA. One of its most worrisome side effects is bladder irritation which can lead to bleeding. Because of this, it is given with a protective agent called Mesna. Mesna can be taken orally or by IV, but it can cause significant nausea. Ifosfamide can also affect blood counts and, in older patients, can cause confusion or delirium.

In these cases, disease that does not respond to second-line treatment is a very worrisome situation and it is not likely that further treatment will be any more effective. A careful and balanced discussion on potential benefits and the probable side effects of further treatment is absolutely necessary.

Joan said:

You do want to ask your doctors if the treatments you receive the first time around will compromise what can be done if the cancer recurs. It is another of the weigh-in factors that

*you should know when you are making the original deci-
sions for your treatment.*

68. What is a clinical trial?

A clinical trial is a study of a new treatment. There are
rigorous guidelines and principles that govern clinical
research in people, which are designed to ensure the
scientific merit of the study, patient safety, and patient
independence (or autonomy).

First, all clinical trials must be reviewed before they can
be offered to patients. This review occurs at the institutional level by the Institutional Review Board (IRB).
They are tasked with making sure the protocol makes
scientific sense, that a safety plan is in place, and that
patient information will be kept confidential. If the federal government is funding the protocol, then a review
must occur at the National Cancer Institute as well.
If the trial is being sponsored by industry (i.e., a new
drug trial sponsored by the makers of that drug), then
industry review will occur before it can go to institutions.
In all cases, the various reviews run independent of the
others. In fact, an important function of the IRB is to
make sure that any relationship between the study per-
sonnel at the institution (the doctors, nurses, research
aides) and sponsor of the study is disclosed before the
study opens. If a conflict of interest exists, the IRB
reserves the right not to open the study to enrollment,
or else mandate that all patients are informed of the
relationship between study staff and trial.

Second, all trials require your informed consent. This is
more than just signing a piece of paper. It is a document
mandated by the federal government that explains, in
language that non-medical people should understand,
the entire study: what question is being asked, what

treatment is being tried, potential side effects of treatment, how long the study will be, and your alternatives if you choose not to do it. It is the only documentation that will exist to prove that you elected to participate in the trial, and you should be provided a copy of the consent form.

Finally, all treatment on trial requires your agreement to proceed. Any trial can be stopped at any time and you can make this call if you find the study is not right for you, for whatever reason. No one can make you do or continue a study. The biggest difference between a person on a trial and a common lab rat is that very power you never give up—on or off a study: your ability to decide what's right for you.

Any trial can be stopped at any time and you can make this call if you find the study is not right for you, for whatever reason.

69. Are there different types of clinical trials?

In oncology, three major trial types are performed. The first is the phase I trial. This is usually the first experience an oncologist will have with patients, and is also referred to as a "first in humans" type of study. As such, investigators usually don't have a clear idea of what dose a drug should be given at, what schedule it should be administered on (i.e., weekly, daily, every three weeks), and what side effects can be expected. It is important to realize that phase I trials are not designed to test how active a drug is.

In these studies, a drug may undergo various levels of testing, commonly referred to as dose-levels. Patients are assigned to treatment at a specific dose level and then followed for any side effects. If that dose level is clinically safe (i.e., no dangerous or worrisome side effects are seen), then the next dose level would be opened to patients, and so on. This would go on until a certain number of side effects are seen. That dose

Maximal tolerated dose

In clinical trials, the dose level where serious side effects emerge.

level where serious side effects emerge is deemed the **maximal tolerated dose** and further testing may be recommended at the dose level that preceded it. Another function of the phase I trial is to better understand how the body processes the new treatment. This may result in a very significant time commitment on your part, as investigators may ask you to do repeated blood testing or radiology tests, all in a better effort to understand the effects of the drug.

Once the phase I trials have been completed, a phase II trial is opened. The phase II objective is to document how well the drug works. Usually, the study will be restricted to a very specific population—open only to women who have recurrent endometrial cancer but who have never received chemotherapy before. The purpose of this is to study as similar a population as possible so that activity can be defined. One could imagine that if a study enrolled all comers regardless of type (so, enrolled sarcomas and adenocarcinomas), but was designed to test activity, the drug may not look very good. Some phase II studies are done in stages. This will avoid exposing patients to an inactive treatment. In these phase II studies, a certain number of patients are enrolled in the first stage. Once enrolled, the study would close until the activity of the drug in this first group was determined. If it looked encouraging, then the second stage would enroll and study would be completed. If the activity in the first stage did not look at all promising, the study would end and no further patients would be exposed to what was ultimately an inactive treatment.

Phase III studies are opened only if the activity in phase II appears very promising. These studies are often used to help register the drug with the Food and Drug

Administration (FDA) so it can be approved for use. Phase III trials are also called randomized clinical trials. In these studies, the experimental treatment is being directly compared to standard of care, with the aim of learning whether experimental treatment improves on what is currently available. In most cases, improvement is measured by survival: how much longer did patients receiving experimental treatment live without disease getting worse (progression-free survival) or stay alive (overall survival). Patients on these studies do not get to choose their treatment; rather, they are assigned in random fashion to either treatment. In most cases, even the doctor is not aware of which treatment is being given. However, the data from phase III trials help us to improve on the options for people living with cancer.

Sometimes a drug appears so promising that patients ask for it off trials. These may be available on compassionate use programs. These programs are set up by the drug manufacturer to provide access to patients off a specific treatment trial. It is a highly regulated program that still requires permission from the institution or hospital before it can be done. Oftentimes, single patient clinical trial applications to the IRB are required before compassionate use can be given.

70. When should I consider a clinical trial?

This is a very personal decision without a right answer. Investigators are interested in improving treatments for women with endometrial cancer across the spectrum: from how best to treat newly diagnosed disease to finding new treatments for women living with recurrent disease. Currently, there are trials in the post-operative treatment of women with newly diagnosed endometrial cancer, medical treatment of uterine sarcomas, and the second-line treatment of endometrial cancer. So, the best answer

You should consider a clinical trial no matter where you happen to be in your life as a uterine cancer survivor.

is that you should consider a clinical trial no matter where you happen to be in your life as a uterine cancer survivor.

Among the questions in current trials right now are the following:

1. What is the best treatment of endometrial adenocarcinomas after surgery? We are looking at ways to combine radiation and chemotherapy and the use of full-dose chemotherapy with the aim of improving survival. Prior studies have shown that chemotherapy is more effective than radiation in the post-surgical treatment of endometrial cancer. However, the way the disease comes back is different. In women treated with radiation, disease tends to come back in the lungs. For those treated with chemotherapy, it comes back in the pelvis. Researchers are looking for ways to combine these regimens to hopefully reduce the risk for cancer returns both locally and at distant sites.

2. What is the best treatment for uterine sarcomas? Even today we do not know the best way to approach uterine sarcomas. Current trials are looking for the best combination of drugs and the best sequence of drugs with an aim to reduce the risk that sarcomas will return.

3. For women who have recurred after chemotherapy, what is the best treatment? Given the lack of effective strategies, a lot of work is going into the evaluation of potentially new agents with activity. Among the drugs that appear promising are:
   • bevacizumab (which blocks the formation of new blood vessels on tumors, leading them to starve)
   • ixabepilone (a drug that acts like paclitaxel to block cells from dividing)
   • a class of drugs called mTOR inhibitors (which stands for mammalian targets of rapamycin)

The major group that conducts trials in uterine cancers is the Gynecologic Oncology Group. This is a national group comprised of participants from hospitals and oncology practices located across the country that are dedicated to research in female tract cancers. They are constantly developing, running, and analyzing clinical trials. They also have a highly specialized infrastructure that allows them to systematically test drugs for activity. For more information, visit their website (listed in Question 100).

Joan said:

There was not a clinical trial available for me but I did do a lot of thinking about this before I knew that. My cancer was diagnosed incrementally with the grade getting successively worse and worse. I found, while I wanted to be aggressive about my treatment after surgery, I was not a candidate for early-stage trials. My personality wasn't one to gamble on an unknown. I think I may have joined a Phase III trial but one wasn't available so I don't know for sure.

PART EIGHT

Treatment at the End of Life

How will I know when I am terminal?

What do I tell my family?

What does hospice mean?

More . . .

71. How do women die from uterine cancer?

Women with uterine cancer tend to die from metastatic disease. Sometimes the disease will spread in the abdomen and close off the bowels, preventing you from eating and causing you to vomit anything that you attempt to eat. It can also cause significant pain as the bowels stretch due to the cancer overlying it, called a bowel obstruction, and this constellation of symptoms can herald the end of life. Other times, the cancer can overwhelm the body and cause profound weakness, difficulty breathing, and pain. In the process of trying to control pain, the weakness can worsen and women at the end of their lives may spend much of their day asleep rather than awake or active. These also can herald the end of one's life.

72. How will I know when I am terminal?

Predicting when someone enters the final phase is very difficult, but certain signs are present that can help you and your doctor to determine this. If you have been through a number of treatments and the cancer continues to grow or does not otherwise respond to treatment, it is not likely that further treatment will help. In addition, if pain increases, weakness worsens, or you are not able to eat, all of these are worrisome signs that the cancer cannot be medically controlled. More importantly, however, the acknowledgment that you are entering a terminal phase in your care requires an open relationship between you and your doctor paved in honesty and trust.

73. What is a PEG tube?

PEG stands for **percutaneous endoscopic gastrostomy**. It is essentially a tube that is placed by a gastrointestinal (GI) specialist in an outpatient procedure. In the context of a chronic bowel obstruction, the purpose of a

If you have been through a number of treatments and the cancer continues to grow or does not otherwise respond to treatment, it is not likely that further treatment will help.

Percutaneous endoscopic gastrostomy (PEG)

A tube placed by a gastrointestinal (GI) specialist in an outpatient procedure. In the context of a chronic bowel obstruction, the purpose of a PEG tube is to provide an alternative way for fluid to go, instead of vomiting to provide relief for the woman who has a chronic bowel obstruction.

PEG tube is to provide an alternative way for fluid to go, instead of vomiting. A PEG is placed during an outpatient procedure that requires the patient to be sedated. The endoscope, which is a very small camera housed in a fiber optic tube, is passed through your mouth and down your esophagus into the stomach. Given the light that is found in the endoscope, the GI doctor can see it through the abdominal wall. Once it is visualized, a needle is passed from the outside into the patient's abdomen and eventually into the stomach, where a suture is then attached to the needle and taken up via the endoscope and tied to the PEG tube. The procedure is repeated and the PEG tube travels from the outside, through the mouth and esophagus, into the stomach and eventually through the abdominal wall. Once in place, a balloon is inflated in the stomach to anchor the tube in place.

The PEG tube can provide relief for the woman who has a chronic bowel obstruction. Unfortunately, since the bowels are not functional, it cannot be used for nutrition. It is simply a comfort measure at the end of life.

74. What is TPN?

TPN stands for **total parenteral nutrition**. It is sometimes considered in women whose bowels no longer work. The objective is to provide the patient with nutrition at the end of life, so that she does not starve to death.

However, TPN often can cause more problems than it can help. TPN rarely will prolong the life of a patient with end-stage cancer. It is thought that the TPN does not really provide nutrition to the patient, but rather serves as a source of nutrition for the cancer. In addition, as the body weakens, less protein is being made. TPN can, unfortunately, result in a huge fluid shift into the soft tissue (called **third spacing**) and can result in

Total parenteral nutrition (TPN)
A method used to provide the patient whose bowels no longer work with nutrition at the end of life, so that she does not starve to death.

Third spacing
Fluid shift into the soft tissue, sometimes caused by TPN.

85

Nidus

A central point or locus of an infection.

Palliative care

The active management of patients at the end of life in which death is not viewed as something to be avoided, but is embraced as a part of the normal cycle of life.

significant fluid accumulation in the arms, legs, and torso. It is not uncommon for a woman to gain 15–30 pounds of excess fluid weight. In addition, it can serve as a **nidus** for a blood infection. The sugar that is used in the TPN can promote the development of an infection, which can prove fatal. Finally, it can also make the blood thicker, predisposing it to clot formation. Given the pros and cons of TPN, it is often not recommended during the terminal phases of uterine cancer. Still, it is a situation that will vary for each woman, and a discussion between your doctor and you is essential if it comes to this.

75. What does palliative care mean?

Palliative care is the active management of patients at the end of life. With palliative care, death is not viewed as something to be avoided, but is embraced as a part of the normal cycle of life. The aim of care at this phase is to help those who are sick remain as active as possible for as long as possible. It also is designed to manage the symptoms that can be present when a woman is at the end of her life, including active management of pain, nausea and vomiting, and tiredness. Even more than this, it is meant to address all of the issues that can accompany the end of life, including issues related to religion, fear, depression, and the other psychological and spiritual aspects of care. Finally, palliative care embraces the family and social supports of the woman with end-stage cancer to assist them as they help their loved one and to help them cope in what is often a very difficult time.

The aim of care at this phase is to help those who are sick remain as active as possible for as long as possible.

76. What do I tell my family?

Your family and friends can be a source of strength and support for you. It is important that you allow them to help you if they offer to do so because no one should go through cancer alone. Part of this is keeping them as involved as you feel comfortable and letting them know where you are in your cancer journey. If things do not look good and the cancer appears to be "taking over," your support system can help you adjust to emotionally and physically hard times. Many doctors recommend appropriate honesty to their patients, encouraging them to let those who love them (and whom they in turn love) participate in their care as much as they are willing to, and as much as the patient wants them to.

77. What is a living will? What about a health care proxy?

Both a living will and a health care proxy are components of Advance Care Planning. A living will is a legal document that covers the types of treatment you wish for yourself. They are instructions that can be followed by your doctors and caregivers if you are not able to participate in your care. They can encompass directions related to intensive care, artificial nutrition, the use of IV fluids, and artificial life support. The living will speaks for you in the event you no longer can and these wishes are often delivered by whomever you name your health care proxy. The health care proxy is a legally named person to whom you have given the power to make decisions in case you are not able to. It may be your spouse, child, best friend, or lover, but in any case, it is important that someone you trust be named, hopefully before he or she is needed, so you both can discuss these very important health-related issues.

Joan said:

I talked with my family before my hysterectomy so I could have a living will and a health care proxy on file with all my doctors and the hospital prior to my surgery. These are things we all should have along with a standard will. However, it is human nature to put off thinking and doing anything about them . . . cancer brings it to the forefront.

78. What does hospice mean?

Hospice is otherwise termed end-of-life care. When treatments are no longer working and a woman becomes very sick because of her cancer, her doctor may recommend hospice. It represents a concerted effort by doctors and other health care providers to recognize that the end of life is a part of the disease process. Medical professionals have a responsibility to help the patient and her family to remain as comfortable as possible, with dignity and free of pain. Hospice care can be delivered either in an inpatient facility (either a hospital or nursing home-type setting) or at home. The overarching goal of hospice is to ensure that women with end-stage cancer die with dignity and in peace. It should not be taken to mean that your physicians are "giving up" on you. Instead, it should be viewed as an acknowledgment that a patient is entering the final phase of her life, and instead of active treatment, active care is undertaken aimed at improving each hour and each day for her and her loved ones.

The overarching goal of hospice is to ensure that women with end-stage cancer die with dignity and in peace.

79. What does DNR stand for?

DNR stands for "do not resuscitate." This order represents your wishes in case something happens to you that without the use of machines, you would likely die. If you were unable to speak for yourself, these wishes will help your family, your physician, or your health care proxy to make decisions for you when that time comes. In a DNR order, you would be asked to state specifically what you would want done and what you would not want done if you were to have a life-threatening event.

These decisions are, in large part, state determined. For example, in Connecticut, a DNR order must specify clearly if you do or do not want to have a tube inserted into your throat to help you breathe (**intubation**), cardiac resuscitation, intravenous fluids, or total parenteral nutrition (TPN). In New York, both intubation and cardiac resuscitation are included in the DNR order.

Intubation

A tube inserted into a patient's throat to help her breathe.

You should not wait to establish a DNR order until you become so sick that you have to make the decision without having time to really think about it or until you are considered terminal. The best time to discuss it is when you are still healthy, so that you and your family can ask questions and thoroughly talk it over with your doctor.

It's important to realize that a DNR order is not permanent. If, at any point, you change your mind regarding what you would want for yourself in a life-threatening situation, your health care team and your family must respect your wishes.

Treatment at the End of Life

PART NINE

Survivorship Issues for Women with Uterine Cancer

What causes pain for women with uterine cancer?

Will my sex life be affected after I complete my uterine cancer treatment?

How can I cope with uterine cancer?

More . . .

80. I am on chemotherapy. What kind of precautions do I need to take?

Chemotherapy will decrease your body's ability to fight infections and may also decrease your red blood cell count, which will result in anemia. Women on chemotherapy must be careful to stay away from large crowds of people or people who are sick during the time when their infection cell counts are low, usually about 5–10 days after treatment.

Chemotherapy may also cause neuropathy, or tingling in your fingers and toes. You must pay careful attention to these symptoms and report them to your doctor if they occur. Some kinds of chemotherapy can cause skin problems, which must also be reported to your doctor.

The medications that are used to combat nausea during chemotherapy can cause significant constipation. Be aware of this and make sure to keep bowel function carefully under control with stool softeners and diet modification as needed. Make sure you call your doctor if you have not had a bowel movement for three days or if you have significant abdominal pain.

The medications that are used to avoid allergic reaction to chemotherapy can increase blood sugar levels. If you are a diabetic you must be very careful to monitor your blood sugars carefully around the time of your chemotherapy.

Pain

81. What causes pain for women with uterine cancer?

Women can have pain related to surgery; this normally lasts 2–4 weeks after surgery. This pain is treated with narcotic medications that are then slowly tapered off and exchanged for ibuprofen or Tylenol as the woman heals.

Women on chemotherapy must be careful to stay away from large crowds of people or people who are sick during the time when their infection cell counts are low.

Recurrent disease can cause pain but most often does not. Recurrence of disease at the top of the vagina usually results in painless bleeding. A lymph node recurrence may also be asymptomatic, but sometimes a lymph node recurrence can result in back or abdominal pain and this should be reported to your doctor. A bone metastasis is unusual, but if it occurs would result in bony pain.

Sometimes pain in the abdomen can occur as a result of bowel obstruction. Bowel obstructions can be caused by surgical adhesions or scar tissue, and are more likely to occur if the woman has received treatment with post-operative radiation therapy. A bowel obstruction can be diagnosed by an abdominal series or CT scan and usually must be repaired surgically.

Pain in the pelvis can result from lymphocysts, which are collections of lymphatic fluid that occur after lymph node dissection. These lymphocysts are most often painless and will resolve on their own; if the woman is having pain, the lymphocysts can be drained with a needle with guidance from a CT scan.

82. What should I do to manage pain?

Make sure that you discuss pain with your doctor to be sure that your pain is what is normally expected after surgery. Surgical pain can be managed either with narcotic medication or ibuprofen or Tylenol.

Pain that is caused by other problems needs to be managed by identifying and managing the underlying problem.

Cancer-related pain often requires a multi-tiered approach, much like treating a fire. One works to put out the flame, but then must ensure the embers do not re-ignite.

This is often managed acutely by using quick acting pain medications. Opiates can be administered IV for immediate relief, and if the pain is constant and severe, can be administered by continuous infusion using patient-controlled anesthesia (PCA) pumps, which release a safe dose hourly, and allow rescue doses as well. In most cases this requires hospitalization, though it can be made available at home for patients whose pain has proven to be quite difficult to control.

Once controlled, short acting drugs are converted into longer acting drugs, which are available by mouth or as a patch. The dose can be determined by how much IV medication you used to get you out of pain, and provide the source of medications that allows you to also leave the hospital.

Targeting the inflammatory response, which often worsens or triggers worse pain, is also required. This can be achieved by around-the-clock use of acetaminophen or non-steroidal anti-inflammatory drugs.

For medications and dosing of the various agents, it is best to speak to your doctor.

Joan said:

Keep a daily diary (I use my daytimer from work) to list your daily aches and pains. Tell your doctor about all of them—or better yet, give him a print out. It is extremely important that they have all the information of your reactions and side effects—both during and after treatments.

I have also taken advantage of acupuncture and massages that are available through the oncology department I am being treated by. I figure it's wise to be open to all types of care. I have found the acupuncture especially has been a help with the aches and pains, nausea and fatigue.

Fertility and Parenting

83. Are there options if I want to have children in the future?

Sometimes women under 40 will develop endometrial cancer. These women may want to preserve fertility. In certain cases, this may be safe, though there is a risk of tumor progression or recurrence. Women who have grade I endometrioid adenocarcinoma can be considered for treatment that will preserve fertility. These women should be treated by Gynecologic Oncologists. An ultrasound or MRI, or both, will be obtained to be as sure as possible that there is no invasion into the underlying muscle, no involvement of lymph nodes, and no involvement of the tubes and ovaries. A dilatation and curettage is usually performed to confirm the grade of tumor and to be sure that the endometrium is completely removed. If the tumor is confirmed to be grade I and there is no evidence of spread outside of the uterus or invasion into the muscle, the woman may choose to be treated with progesterone to "reverse" the cancer. She must undergo a repeat endometrial biopsy, usually after three months of treatment, to be sure the cancer has reversed. Because the cancer can then recur, she must either (1) continue treatment indefinitely or (2) achieve pregnancy. There have been reported cases of spread of endometrial cancer during or after this kind of treatment, as well as endometrial cancer during pregnancy.

Alternatively, the woman may decide to have her uterus removed, but preserve her ovaries temporarily for the purpose of egg retrieval and embryo freezing. Another woman called a "surrogate" can then carry the embryos to term. The ovaries must be uninvolved with tumor and they are usually removed following the egg retrieval.

If you had your ovaries removed, however, an egg donor will be required in addition to a surrogate.

In a traditional surrogacy agreement, the woman donating her eggs also carries the child. In a gestational surrogacy agreement, the egg donor and the woman carrying the pregnancy are different women. Egg donors can be known or anonymous and are frequently young women. They must be screened psychologically and medically to ensure they understand what egg donation entails and to ensure that they are healthy and free of sexually transmitted diseases. Women looking into becoming surrogates also undergo both mental health and medical screening to ensure they are psychologically and physically prepared to carry a pregnancy. In addition, surrogacy laws vary by state, so using an attorney to assist in legal arrangements is important.

84. What about adoption? Is this also an option?

Recognizing that the pathway to adoption can be a long and winding road is important, as is finding a strong support system including your friends, family, and adoption specialists.

Yes, adoption is another option for prospective parents. Most adoption agencies do not rule out cancer survivors as parents, but do require full disclosure of your medical history and recent medical examinations. Others may require your oncologist to write a letter of support and a declaration that you are cancer free; still others may require you to be cancer free at least five years before considering you as a potential parent. It is important that you work with specialists in the adoption arena who have a good record of working with cancer survivors. Adoption can also take a significant amount of time and effort, leading to psychological and emotional stress. Recognizing that the pathway to adoption can be a long and winding road is important, as is finding a strong support system including your friends, family, and adoption specialists.

Sexual Health

85. What will happen to me with respect to my sexuality after I have my hysterectomy?

The impact of hysterectomy on sexual function is very controversial. While some experts suggest that the uterus does contribute to the female orgasm, these results are contradicted by other work suggesting that hysterectomy can actually relieve **dyspareunia** and has no effect on either the ability to orgasm or on a woman's libido. What is clear is that the satisfaction a woman and her partner had prior to surgery as it relates to sex and well-being directly predicts what sex will be like after surgery, and indirectly, can predict what the response of your partner will be with sex following a hysterectomy. In general, most male partners cannot detect a difference unless the patient makes it obvious.

Dyspareunia

Painful sexual intercourse, due to medical or psychological causes.

All of this supports the notion that a woman's sexuality stems from more than anatomy—that it is a complicated interplay of interpersonal, self-defined, psychological, and physical factors.

Physical changes are unlikely related to a hysterectomy. However, for the premenopausal woman, loss of ovarian function due to **oophorectomy** may result in changes physiologically (which then cause hot flashes and emotional changes) and physically. The loss of estrogen from the ovaries can cause some small degree of hair growth but, in the absence of testosterone supplements, it is not correct to think you will become overly masculinized.

Physical changes are unlikely related to a hysterectomy.

Oophorectomy

Surgical removal of one or both ovaries.

86. Will my sex life be affected after I complete my uterine cancer treatment?

A variety of factors can interfere with a woman's sexuality and sex life. In addition to her psychological make-up and past experience with intimate relationships and medications, cancer treatments may affect how a woman may respond sexually. As we discussed in Question 85, removal of the uterus, ovaries, cervix, and perhaps part of the vagina, may affect your self-esteem and influence how you view yourself as a woman. With extensive surgical resection and radical surgery, women may mourn the loss of their youthful body and femininity. Large tumor resections that involve extensive physical changes, such as bowel removal, may result in functional changes such as **ileostomies**, **colonostomies**, and **ileoconduits** that may be perceived as embarrassing or ugly. Surgical scarring after procedures may interfere with extremity mobility, and even determining a comfortable sexual position may be challenging.

Ileostomy

A surgical opening constructed by bringing the end or loop of small intestine (the ileum) out onto the surface of the skin.

Colonostomy

A surgical operation that creates an opening from the colon to the surface of the body to function as an anus.

Ileoconduit

A small urine reservoir that is surgically created from a segment of bowel.

Still, most women will find that their sex life is not adversely affected after hysterectomy alone. For most women undergoing surgery for uterine cancer, the vagina will be the same and should feel the same to your partner. Removal of your ovaries, however, may change your sex life. If you were premenopausal at the time of your ovary removal, you will note new symptoms of hot flashes and vaginal dryness that you did not experience before your surgery. Both pre- and post-menopausal women may notice a decrease in libido, or sexual desire, after removal of the ovaries.

Some of these symptoms can be treated. Vaginal dryness can be treated with water-based lubricants. Some patients with endometrial cancer can use low-dose estrogen treatment in the vagina to help with dryness; this treatment requires approval from your doctor and a prescription. Sexual desire is a more difficult problem to treat. Testosterone is sometimes used to increase libido but a recent trial in female cancer survivors showed it worked no better than placebo.

Radiation treatment may affect your sex life, particularly if you receive intra-vaginal treatment or brachytherapy. Brachytherapy can cause vaginal scarring and if you do not have intercourse or use a vaginal dilator, the vagina can scar closed. This can seriously impact a woman's capacity for penetrative intercourse and affect her genital pelvic and perhaps her clitoral sensitivity. Sexual sensation or orgasms may be less intense than before, so it may take longer to reach the same level of excitement and arousal. You may be instructed and encouraged to use vaginal dilators as part of your postoperative care plan to maintain vaginal length and integrity. Continued use of dilators with consistent follow-up with a sexual health care provider can help maintain the capacity for vaginal intercourse. In addition to sexual health, maintaining vaginal health is medically important for follow-up, as your doctor will need to examine your vagina and monitor for disease recurrence.

Chemotherapy can cause nausea, diarrhea, or membrane irritation, and can induce premature menopause, which can present as hot flashes and vaginal dryness or atrophy. Loss of hair on the head, eyebrows, eyelashes, and genitals is distressing and affects a female's perception of sexual attractiveness. Chemotherapy-induced early ovarian failure causes menopausal symptoms like hot flashes, sleep problems, vaginal dryness, and mood problems. Vaginal dryness can become a serious medical concern and often leads to painful intercourse on penetration.

87. Sex is painful. What can I do about it?

Painful sex is usually due to vaginal dryness as a result of surgical menopause. Water-based lubricants are safe to use to help this problem. In some cases, your doctor may feel that vaginal estrogen is safe for you to use.

It may be helpful to try sexual intimacy when pain is at a low level with minimal fatigue.

It may be helpful to try sexual intimacy when pain is at a low level with minimal fatigue. Techniques such as warm soaks and physical therapy can help loosen tense muscles. Guided imagery, meditation, deep-muscle relaxation, and avoidance of exhaustion are options that should also be explored. Specifically trained pain management specialists can be consulted to adjust or reduce opioid regimens and add adjunctive or alternative analgesics to lessen fatigue while maintaining sufficient pain relief. Finally, communication with your partner about your pain is very important. Making sure that you are relaxed and ready for sexual intercourse will help decrease discomfort. You may also want to check with your doctor and make sure a urinary tract infection is not causing your symptoms.

88. Will changing what and how I eat improve my sex life?

Although patients try many different foods, such as chocolate, ginseng, oysters, and popular sexual-enhancing diets to facilitate improved sexual function, none has been shown in randomized clinical trials to be beneficial for correcting female sexual complaints. Still, eating right can help you attain an overall sense of well being and if you feel better from how you eat, it might help you improve your body image and as a result, regain an interest in sex.

89. I have absolutely no interest in sex since treatment ended. Can I do anything about it?

Beyond estrogen replacement, there are medications that may lessen the distress of sexual complaints. However, none is FDA approved and there is minimal good scientific data that demonstrate efficacy. However, some of the latest medications include Bupropion, which is an antidepressant with the least sexual side effects. Precautions include insomnia, nervousness, and mild-to-moderate increases in blood pressure as well as a risk of lowering seizure threshold.

Several new drugs are being investigated for specific use in women with low desire. Flibanserin is a new drug being investigated for low female sexual desire. Some of the side effects include nausea, dizziness, fatigue, sleeplessness, and increased bleeding if you are already taking aspirin or an anti-inflammatory drug. Bremelanotide is another drug that acts on a specific protein called the melanocortin receptor. It is in trials specifically in premenopausal women diagnosed with female sexual dysfunction (FSD).

Before considering any of these medications, it is crucial to discuss their potential benefits and risks with your oncologist or clinician.

Hot Flashes

90. What can I do about hot flashes?

Many cancer patients who were pre- or perimenopausal at diagnosis go through abrupt menopause following surgery for uterine cancer. **Chemical menopause** occurs when the woman has received chemicals (like chemotherapy) or medications that temporarily or permanently stop her cycles. **Surgical menopause** is when both ovaries are removed so hormones are no longer produced. There is a grouping of symptoms that often accompany menopause, and the most troublesome include hot flashes and vaginal dryness.

The exact reason and cause for hot flashes is not yet known. However, some researchers think that a hormone

Chemical menopause

Condition that occurs when a woman has received chemicals (like chemotherapy) or medications that temporarily or permanently stop her cycles.

Surgical menopause

When both ovaries are removed so hormones are no longer produced.

called luteinizing hormone (LH) is released at the same time as the levels of estrogen decrease. This release of LH may effect changes such as in veins getting larger, which may cause skin flushing, increased sweating with increased blood flow, increased body temperature, and a rapid heart rate. Some women feel as if they are perspiring, soaking through their clothing.

Each woman's experience with hot flashes is, of course, unique and many women experience hot flashes that are not bothersome and do not warrant therapy. Others are debilitated and cannot function on a day-to-day basis because of their severe menopausal syndrome. Quality-of-life issues are paramount and each woman must decide for herself if her hot flashes need therapy. There are many different methods to treat hot flashes and each woman should decide what is best and safest for her. It is always best to consult with your health care team about your symptoms and which treatment option is best for you specifically.

Hormonal therapy is the mainstay treatment for hot flashes and it remains an effective treatment for troublesome hot flashes. In Question 91 we will discuss this more fully. The North American Menopause Society advocates that only severe and debilitating hot flashes be treated and, if hormones are to be used, one should be using the lowest doses for the shortest amount of time for hot flash and other symptom relief.

Bioidentical hormones

Plant-derived hormones that are created, mixed, and packaged by a pharmacist

Recent media reports advocate compounded **bioidentical hormones** as a safe alternative to hormone replacement therapy. These are plant-derived hormones that are created, mixed, and packaged by a pharmacist who can customize the product according to the physician's specifications. However, according to the American College of Obstetricians and Gynecologists, most compounded products have not undergone strict scientific study and there may be concerns about safety, purity, and efficacy of these products. For this reason, bioidentical hormones are not safer than those prescribed by your doctor. If you are considering taking bioidentical hormones or are now taking a prescribed compound, it may be dangerous for your continued health. It is strongly recommended that you discuss the risks of bioidentical hormones with your cancer specialist and gynecologist.

Even though it may be safe for most endometrial cancer patients to use estrogen alone, many choose not to use these products because of personal choice or fear of developing breast cancer or another type of hormonally-sensitive cancer.

If you are considering taking bioidentical hormones or are now taking a prescribed compound, it may be dangerous for your continued health.

There are a variety of methods to decrease the severity and intensity of hot flashes. Some include environmental changes like wearing absorbent, cotton clothing or dressing in layers so that the outermost layers can be removed when you get a hot flash. In addition, there is specially-designed sleepwear that has been developed for those with nighttime hot flashes and sweats. Cooling techniques such as drinking an ice-cold glass of water, putting a cold moist compress on your face, and using a misting-type spray bottle can help you feel cooler in the middle of a flash. Lowering the thermostat or placing a fan near where you sleep may help. Biofeedback techniques and relaxation techniques like yoga, meditation, and tai chi may also be helpful for troublesome hot flashes. Additionally, regular exercise, avoiding cigarette smoking, and hot baths also can be helpful.

Sometimes changes in diet can help with hot flashes. It may mean avoiding certain triggers like caffeine, alcohol (including beer, wine, and liquor), and spicy foods. Vitamin supplements such as vitamin B_6 (200 or 250 mg daily) or Peridin C (two tablets three times a day) may provide some relief, though it is important not to abandon them too early. Try one supplement at a time for a 4–6 week course. It is also best to review the supplements you choose to take with your oncologist.

Acupuncture is the ancient Chinese medical system where very thin needles are painlessly and strategically placed into the skin. It is used to help control chronic pain, in addition to healing a wide variety of other ailments. Acupuncture works by stimulating specific portions of the nervous system, relieving pain by causing signal transmitters and hormones in the brain to work in different ways. Many women report relief from hot flashes with acupuncture.

Sometimes, prescription medications such as antihypertensive medications and antidepressants can be prescribed to help minimize hot flashes. Antiepileptics like gabapententin also may be effective pharmacological therapy for the hot-flash sufferer; however, they do have some common side effects. It is always important to talk with your doctor or nurse about your medications to see if you should try another type of medicine and to discuss possible side effects. Remember that all medications have some side effects so, in addition to discussing this with your clinician, it is best to carefully read the package insert that comes with the prescription.

91. Do I have *to take hormones after my surgery?*

Following surgery (particularly if the ovaries were removed), you may experience changes related to menopause which, in addition to hot flashes, include vaginal thinning and dryness and chafing during intercourse, to name a few. If symptoms such as these come about, then the use of very low dose estrogen preparations may be very helpful. Hormonal therapy with estrogen is the mainstay treatment for hot flashes. There are many new and effective low-dose preparations that come in all forms of delivery systems including a patch which is placed on your skin in differing areas, rings that can be placed within the vagina, gels that can be applied to the body, vaginal tablets, creams, and other formulations. Every woman should carefully educate herself and analyze the risks and benefits of taking hormones, especially with regard to their symptoms and family and personal history. It is important to discuss your concerns regarding hormones with your doctor.

If you do decide to take hormones, continue to have your physical examinations, clinical breast examination, and annual mammogram. Breast self-examinations and a risk assessment also should be done on a regular basis. If any of your close family members, including sisters, mother, aunts, or other close relatives develop cancers, discuss your continuation on the hormones with your doctor. It is important to report any side effects like abnormal vaginal bleeding to your doctor.

92. Can I take hormone replacement therapy?

As we touched on previously, estrogen has many effects on the genital system. It promotes cell maturation and proliferation and increases blood flow, but it also stimulates secretions. A decrease of estrogen causes decreased blood supply to the genitals, increased dryness, and can lead to painful intercourse and possibly a reactive lowered desire. The use of local vaginal estrogen (creams, rings, and tablets) for the treatment of vaginal atrophy is available and widely accepted. Many products are minimally absorbed, such as estrogen vaginal tablets or estrogen rings. Cream preparations can provide relief from irritation of the pelvic areas, including the vagina and vulva.

Some sexual health providers prefer to prescribe minimally-absorbed local 17β-estradiol tablets, which are minimally absorbed into the systemic circulation. It is important to recognize that estrogen use is not without risks or complications. Some of the side effects include possible blood clots (**thromboembolic events**) and increased heart problems (cardiovascular events). Interestingly, in a large study called the Women's Health Initiative, women taking estrogen only because they had undergone a hysterectomy did not experience an increased risk of breast cancer. Still, that study excluded women with a history of endometrial cancer, so discussing the pros and cons of hormone replacement therapy requires a balanced discussion between you and your doctor.

There is a theoretical risk that taking estrogen will increase the risk of recurrent endometrial cancer in women with the disease. In fact, the estrogen package insert says that women with endometrial cancer should not take this medication. The Gynecology Oncology Group, a large national group in the United States, did a prospective clinical trial that randomized women with endometrial cancer to receive either estrogen or placebo following hysterectomy. The study closed early and did

Thromboembolic events

Blood clots.

not reach its accrual goal; however, it appeared that taking estrogen did not increase the risk of recurrent cancer in the women who took it. The decision to take estrogen after hysterectomy for endometrial cancer is one that each woman should discuss with her doctor.

Coping

93. When am I considered a cancer survivor?

Survivorship is defined from the time you were first diagnosed. Hence, once you hear the phrase, "you have cancer," you become a survivor. Since so many more women (and men) are surviving their cancer, we have realized as a community how important it is to care for survivors and their needs. Hence, a new field of practice has blossomed, and is known as survivorship medicine.

Survivorship medicine is a field devoted to people who have been diagnosed and treated for cancer. The specific goals survivorship medicine encompasses are prevention and early detection. In addition, it offers support for cancer families to help minimize pain, disability, and psychosocial stressors while promoting and encouraging improved quality of life for the cancer patient. The ultimate aim is to provide you, with the help of your health care provider, with the tools to improve your lifestyle and make active health decisions in how to live your life; it will help you live a healthy, active, and productive life.

It is important to acknowledge that living with a history of cancer really means that you will never be the same person as you were before the time of the cancer diagnosis. For uterine cancer patients, survivorship medicine includes the optimizing of general heath maintenance by preventing the development of secondary

Since so many more women (and men) are surviving their cancer, we have realized as a community how important it is to care for survivors and their needs.

cancers whenever possible, and promoting health and well-being with an emphasis on primary and preventative care. This medical plan will encompass the screening for other cancers and prevention of chronic medical illnesses. It also will help direct you to resources as they become needed. Too often, cancer survivors have had nowhere to turn when they wanted to raise or adopt children, discuss sexual function, or relay concerns about protracted treatment side effects. It is the aim of survivorship specialists to be that link between their oncology-specific care and the rest of their lives.

There is no "right way" to react on being called a cancer survivor. While some women embrace survivorship, others embark on a route of positive thinking and begin tai chi, yoga, meditation, and macrobiotic diets, because some women believe that bringing holistic mental treatments into the forefront of their survivorship experience is paramount, while others primarily focus on getting back to their normal routines and work schedules. Yet others react negatively to being called a survivor and would prefer to leave that aspect of their life behind them, touching upon it only when they see their oncologist. It is important to know that each woman's experience in survivorship is different and you should allow yourself the luxury of feeling the way you feel. Allow yourself the time to adapt to the cancer experience and incorporate it into your way of thinking.

It is important to know that each woman's experience in survivorship is different and you should allow yourself the luxury of feeling the way you feel.

Joan said:

At the moment, I consider myself "surviving cancer" but not a survivor. My head has that five-year cancer-free timeframe embedded for being called a "survivor." It is true that every day upright and smiling is a good day.

94. When will I feel like myself again?

It takes time to feel back to yourself after surgery, even if you have minimally invasive surgery. Your doctor will let you resume normal activity and go back to work at 6–8 weeks post-operatively, but most women do not feel back to themselves until 6 months after surgery. Full surgical healing takes 12 months.

You may have side effects after your surgery that get better with time. These include constipation (usually from the pain medication) and a decreased sensation in your bladder. Other side effects may be longer lasting; these include a numb patch on the front of one or both thighs, and swelling in the feet and lower legs. Most women have a complete return to pre-surgical function by six months after the surgery.

If you have extra treatment with radiation or chemotherapy, you can expect your recovery to be delayed by that treatment. Both radiation and chemotherapy can cause side effects that may last for years. Common problems may be fatigue, difficulties with short-term memory, or numbness and tingling. Speak to your doctor if these persist over a year after completing treatment.

95. Are depression or other psychological issues common after treatment?

It is important to understand your feelings after a cancer diagnosis. If this is impacting your ability to have meaningful relationships or is impacting your ability to maintain social connections, business obligations, or is interfering with your quality of life, then it is possible that you have a medical depression. Some other symptoms of depression include:

- Overwhelming sadness
- Anxiety

- Feelings of guilt
- Loss of interest in usual activities and hobbies
- Inability to concentrate
- Loss of appetite
- Feeling overall slowed mentally and physically
- Suicidality

If you have these feelings or your feelings of isolation and sadness are overwhelming, then you must seek medical and psychological counseling. Depression is a medical illness that requires treatment; do not be scared or fear that you will be judged for your low mood; it is common and many cancer survivors suffer from low mood changes.

96. How can I cope with uterine cancer?

Many different types of integrative care therapies have been helpful when used by cancer patients; some can help keep stress to a minimum and relieve daily anxiety and pressures. Try one or another for a few weeks and see how you feel. If it works, keep with it, if not, then try another type. Some popular therapies are:

- Reflexology: This is the application of pressure to different areas of the foot with the objective of relieving stress and pain.
- Massage: This involves gentle pressure and slow body stretching. Various forms are practiced, including Shiatsu and Swedish techniques.
- Aromatherapy: This uses inhaling specific scents (aromas) to help maintain bodily health. Essential oils are concentrated aromas that can be inhaled to promote a quiet sense of peace. Lavender, rosemary, or chamomile essence can be purchased at the local store; a few drops in bath water can be especially soothing.

- Reiki: This is a form of martial arts and can promote a sense of calmness and tranquility. It may help you to reduce anxiety and maintain an ordered sense of calmness.
- Meditation involves breathing regulation and mind power. Using specific sitting postures and hand positions, you can gain inner calmness and serenity.
- Yoga is a popular exercise that many women use to help tone their bodies and relax their minds. It consists of performing a series of stretching exercises and holding different postures while deeply breathing, which some find quite calming.

Many national cancer centers have post-treatment resource centers and survivorship programs that organize group support programs for female cancer survivors, and they are cancer diagnosis-specific. Share your specific concerns with your health care provider. They may be able to direct you to professional organizations or other health care providers that can help you regain your mental health. It is not something you should be ashamed about; many survivors face the same problems that you are going through, and emotional health is an important facet of your recovery.

Prevention and Screening

97. How are women followed after treatment for uterine cancer?

Women with very early endometrial cancer (grade 1, non-invasive) may be followed every six months for two years and then discharged from the cancer clinic. All other women are followed every three months for two years, then every six months for two years, and then yearly to complete five years of follow-up.

Follow-up consists of full physical examination including pelvic examination. A speculum examination to examine the vaginal lining is very important, but Pap smears are not necessary since the cervix has been removed. There is no role for routine CT scans, but a CT scan should be ordered if a woman is having a new symptom or if there is a new finding on physical examination. CT scans can diagnose enlarged lymph nodes or masses in the abdomen or pelvis that may represent recurrent disease.

If your doctor is concerned about disease recurrence he or she will likely schedule a biopsy to confirm that your disease has recurred.

Beyond cancer-specific follow-up, according to the American College of Obstetricians and Gynecologists' technical bulletin on primary and preventative care on periodic assessment for women, some of the important components of a comprehensive examination include assessments of cardiac health (blood pressure, cholesterol screening), dental examinations, vision examinations, and diabetes screening; medication review of prescribed and over-the-counter medications, herbs and supplements (including vitamins), and prescription medications; tobacco, alcohol, and drug use screening; breast health annual mammography; vaccinations; skin screening, sun health and skin cancer prevention; and sexuality screening. For those of child-bearing potential, reviews of contraception, safer sex practices and condom use, HIV and other sexually transmitted disease screening and prevention are required.

Other areas that should be addressed with the cancer survivor include issues related to nutrition, fitness, and psychosocial well-being by screening for psychiatric illnesses like depression and anxiety, evaluating employment satisfaction and enjoyment, ruling out job burnout and stress, screening for domestic partner abuse (physical, emotional, and sexual), and abuse history (sexual, physical, verbal, and emotional).

The American College of Obstetricians' new patient educational pamphlet published in 2007, entitled *Staying Healthy at All Ages* is a helpful booklet that discusses these issues for women of all ages. Speak with your doctor today about formulating a healthy plan to detect disease early, prevent other cancers, and stay healthy.

Obviously all of these issues can overwhelm both you and your oncologist. This provides the foundation for survivorship medicine and the importance of keeping your primary care providers and oncology providers all aligned to the same goals for your long-term health and well-being.

Joan said:

I know your doctor will have you on a schedule of follow-up visits but one thing I've learned is to listen to my body. I am the only one who knows or will notice the subtle changes that may happen. You have to keep track of what seems different and make sure the doctor understands and listens to you.

98. What should I be screened for? I already had cancer.

Different women are at risk for differing cancers, so it is best to individualize your plan and, just because you had uterine cancer does not mean you are not at risk for others. The bottom line is that your care needs to be tailored to your specific history and your specific medical needs. Your doctor should look inside the vagina at every visit to make sure there is no evidence of cancer recurrence in the vagina (the most common place for endometrial cancer to come back). However, most gynecologic oncologists will not perform a Pap smear. The Pap smear is designed to detect cervical cancer (and your cervix has been removed!) and data suggest that performing a Pap smear does not help to pick up a recurrence of endometrial cancer earlier than just looking at the vagina or waiting for symptoms (usually vaginal bleeding). You should continue to have Pap smears, however, if you have a history of having abnormal Pap smears of your cervix or if you have a history of treatment for cervical pre-cancer, since your vagina is also at risk for developing this same kind of pre-cancer.

Typically your gynecologic oncologist will perform these vaginal examinations for several years after your cancer treatment in order to ensure that you have not had a cancer recurrence. This is done in conjunction with a full physical examination, including listening to your heart and lungs and examining your abdomen. You should tell your gynecologic oncologist of any new problems you may be having, especially abdominal pain or bloating, change in bowel or bladder habits, or vaginal bleeding or discharge.

Cancer of the vulva and clitoris are rather rare and early diagnosis and treatments are needed to prevent extensive spread of the disease. Smoking, HPV infection, multiple sexual partners, HIV infection, or a history of cervical abnormalities all may contribute to the development of vulvar cancer. Because there is no recommended screening test to detect vulvar or clitoral cancer, it is important to note if you have any unusual symptoms including itchiness, burning in the vulvar area, dry scaly skin changes or bleeding, or abnormal discharge from the vulvar area.

You should report these changes to your doctor and you may need a small outpatient biopsy to get a definitive diagnosis of the troubling area. Many women perform self vulvar examination with the aid of a handheld mirror and report any changes in skin color or changes in surface texture to the doctor.

Ovarian cancer does not have any specific, clear-cut presenting symptoms. Very often, patients present with disease that is advanced in stage and has spread to many pelvic or abdominal organs. Some of the vague symptoms associated with ovarian cancer may be abdominal gas or unexplained bloating that does not go away, pelvic pressure, or a swollen abdomen. Recent research indicates that some women complain of urinary symptoms in the early stages of ovarian cancer. If you are at an increased risk because of your ethnicity, genetic problems, a strong family history for either breast or ovarian cancer, or a personal history of breast cancer before the age of 50, you may be eligible for ovarian cancer screening, but this should only be done as part of a formalized program or clinical trial.

Many women of all races, socioeconomic backgrounds, religions, and social standing will develop breast cancer over the course of their lifetimes, and one in seven women will develop breast cancer in her lifetime. Breast health awareness is important so that you can maintain excellent breast health. Some of the myths concerning breast cancer should be dispelled. At the present time, there are no accurate scientific data that directly link underwire bras, antiperspirant usage, or having had an elective termination of pregnancy with breast cancer. Mammography (a special x-ray of the breast where the radiation exposure of the breast tissue is minimal), clinical breast examination by a physician,

and breast self-examination are three of the best techniques to help detect breast disease at an early stage
and all contribute to excellent breast health.

Recently, the United States Preventive Services Task
Force revised their screening mammography recommendations. They no longer recommended routine mammo-
graphic screening for women under 50; however, those
deemed at an increased risk of developing breast cancer
should start earlier. Such a decision requires that you
speak to your doctor. Still, the advice from the American
Cancer Society remains unchanged; they recommend
that mammograms begin at the age of 40. After that,
mammograms should be repeated every 1 to 2 years until
the age of 50, when they should be done on an annual
basis. Clinical breast examination by a health care professional should be a part of the routine annual health maintenance examination.

On the day of your mammogram, you should not use
deodorant or antiperspirant, because some contain
certain ingredients that can interfere with correct inter-
pretation of the mammogram. You may want to wear a
two-piece outfit, because you will need to be undressed
from the waist up for the mammogram procedure. The
best time to have a mammogram is shortly after your
menstrual cycle. Always follow up and call your gynecologist or health care provider if you do not receive your
mammogram results within a few days after the test.

According to the Cancer Research and Prevention
Foundation, colon cancer is the second leading cause of
cancer deaths in the United States. Close to 145,000
women and men are diagnosed and between 55,000 and
56,000 die each year from the disease. When discovered
early, colon cancer is treatable and often curable. Colon
cancer is a serious medical illness for women and most
medical associations advocate colon screening starting at

the age of 50. There are several methods to screen for colon cancer. Some include a fecal occult blood test for which you will be given a home testing card kit. You are asked to get a sample of stool on the card, insert it into the supplied plastic sleeve, and mail it to a laboratory. The card sample then is tested for the presence or absence of blood. Other tests are a flexible sigmoidoscopy (every five years), colonoscopy, and double-contrast barium enema. It is understandable that you may be fearful or embarrassed about the colon, but you must remember that rectal screening is one of the positive steps you can take toward disease discovery and early effective treatment. A **colonoscopy** is a medical outpatient surgical procedure that is the screening tool to detect colonic abnormalities and precancerous growths in the colon. It looks at the large intestine or colon and rectum. It is the best type of test that can image the lining (colonic mucosa) and can be used to accurately identify colon cancer. After a special preparation that cleanses the colon, a small tube, which is thin and flexible and has a small video camera with a light source at the end, is placed within the rectum and advanced so that the gastrointestinal specialist can see the entire lining of the colon. The tube is lubricated so that it can be advanced into the colon with little discomfort. You will have received some sedation before the procedure, so you will be in a relaxed state of mind called "twilight." You will be conscious but unable to recall all of the details of the procedure.

Sun health is very important to prevent damage from the sun and skin cancer. Limit your exposure to the sun during the times when the sun is the most harmful, from 10 AM to 4 PM; cover the parts of your body exposed to the sun with long-sleeved, lightweight clothing. Seek shade and wear hats that shield your face, ears, head, and neck, and wear eye protection against the sun's damaging rays. Liberal use of a non-expired sunscreen

Colonoscopy

An outpatient surgical procedure that is the screening tool to detect colonic abnormalities and precancerous growths in the colon.

117

that has a minimum sun protection factor (SPF) of 15 and that can block both the UVA and UVB rays of the sun is essential. You should apply a sunscreen often and liberally, on both sunny and cloudy/hazy days. Sunscreens should be applied approximately 30 minutes before exposure to the sun and should be applied repeatedly, especially when engaging in water sports, swimming, or other activities that have caused a lot of perspiration.

99. Does having uterine cancer increase my risk of getting another cancer?

Women with endometrial cancer are potentially at increased risk for other cancers such as breast and colon cancers, especially if anyone in their family has had any of these cancers.

Joan said:

I was worried about this because of a medical condition I've had most of my adult life. It was good to be reassured that there is no correlation to increased risk. While the possibility of future cancer is more near, it is not a given. You cannot live your life with the constant thought of cancer coming back or of another type of cancer diagnosis.

100. Where can I get more information?

There are numerous resources available for you or your loved ones regarding cervical cancer. Fortunately, the Internet has put a significant amount of resources within reach for many women. Some of the more help-ful ones are listed in the Resources section, located at the end of this book.

Joan said:

I utilized www.webmd.com and also the Mayo Clinic website in the beginning for the general information on surgery etc. I then used the Dana Farber Cancer Institute's site when I became associated with their medical staff. Once my complete diagnosis was determined, I became very familiar with the American Cancer Society's site and also the National Cancer Institute.

You have to keep good records of your own treatments and protocols. The doctors you have attending you see many patients every day who are having different/specific treatments. They may not always remember the exact details of your treatment regimen. If they talk about something other than what was previously discussed, stop them and correct them. Ask them why the protocol is being changed—is it new information—newly released studies? Make sure there should be a change and why it is better than what was previously agreed upon.

Resources

About Uterine Cancer

National Cancer Institute: www.cancer.gov/cancertopics/types/
American Cancer Society: www.cancer.org
American Society of Clinical Oncology: www.asco.org
Gynecologic Cancer Foundation: www.thegcf.org
Society of Gynecologic Oncologists: www.sgo.org
Women's Cancer Network: www.wcn.org

Treatment Options

Clinical Trials: www.clinicaltrials.gov
Gynecologic Oncology Group: www.gog.org
National Comprehensive Cancer Network (NCCN): www.nccn.org

Survivorship

National Coalition for Cancer Survivorship: www.canceradvocacy.org
Lance Armstrong Foundation: www.livestrong.org
NCI Office of Cancer Survivorship: http://cancercontrol.cancer.gov/ocs/
    office-survivorship.html

Sexual Health

The Women's Sexual Health Foundation: www.twshf.org
The International Society for the Study of Women's Sexual Health:
    www.isswsh.org
North American Menopause Society: www.menopause.org
Association of Reproductive Health Professionals: www.arhp.org

Fertility

FertileHope: www.fertilehope.org

Glossary

Adenocarcinoma: A form of cancer that arises from the glands.

Adipose: The fat tissue, which is able to store high levels of hormones that can be converted to estrogen and stimulate the endometrium to create endometrial cancer.

Apoptosis: Programmed cell death.

Benign: Non-threatening, non-cancerous.

Bioidentical hormones: Plant-derived hormones that are created, mixed, and packaged by a pharmacist.

Biopsy: Taking a piece of a tumor to determine whether it is malignant or benign.

Brachytherapy: A method of radiation treatment in which the source of radiation is placed close to the surface of the body or within a body cavity (Example: vagina).

Cancer: The end product of cells that no longer follow the usual order of cell growth, division, and death.

Carcinosarcomas: Dual cancers with an epithelial component (carcino-) and the sarcoma component.

Cardiomyopathy: Weakening of the heart muscle causing it not to function well.

Chemical menopause: Condition that occurs when a woman has received chemicals (like chemotherapy) or medications that temporarily or permanently stop her cycles.

Choriocarcinoma: A very aggressive form of GTN that usually develops after a complete mole, but rarely can be seen after a partial mole or even a normal pregnancy.

Clinical trial: A study of a new treatment, following rigorous guidelines and principles that govern clinical research in people, which are designed to ensure the scientific merit of the study, patient safety, and patient independence.

Colonoscopy: An outpatient surgical procedure that is the screening tool to detect colonic abnormalities and pre-cancerous growths in the colon.

Colonostomy: A surgical operation that creates an opening from the colon to the surface of the body to function as an anus.

Complex atypical hyperplasia: A condition of the endometrium which is thought to be a precursor lesion for endometrial adenocarcinoma.

Computed tomography (CT): Test which uses x-rays to build a picture and is sometimes administered in combination with a PET scan to help give both a structural and functional assessment of a tumor.

Corpus: Also called the uterus.

D&C: D&C stands for dilatation and curettage. In this procedure the surgeon will dilate, or open, the cervix in order to perform a curettage, or scraping, of the uterine cavity.

Differentiation: Changes in the cells of developing infants that enable cells to perform different functions.

DNR: Means "do not resuscitate." This order represents the patient's wishes in case she becomes unable to speak for herself.

Dyspareunia: Painful sexual intercourse, due to medical or psychological causes.

Dyspnea on exertion: Shortness of breath during activities like walking, sometimes a side effect of chemotherapy in which the heart muscle is weakened.

Echogenic foci: An area of abnormal signaling on ultrasound.

Endometrial cancer: Cancer of the uterine lining.

Endometrial intraepithelial neoplasia (EIN): Condition thought to be a precursor lesion for uterine serous papillary carcinoma.

Endometrial stromal sarcomas: Cancers which do not arise from the muscle, but from the supporting tissue of the uterus (called the stroma).

Endometrium: Lining of the uterus which becomes thicker when a woman's ovaries are producing estrogen.

Excision: Surgical removal of tissue.

Field: The area of treatment.

Fluorodeoxyglucose positron emission test (FDG-PET): A radiologic study that uses information about the metabolism or activity of tumors to determine the extent a cancer has spread.

Fibroid: A muscular tumor that develops from the wall of the uterus and can develop into the uterine cavity (called a submucosal fibroid), within the wall of the uterus (called an intramural fibroid), or outside of the uterus (subserosal fibroid). They can even develop as an outpouching connected to the uterus by a stalk, much like a mushroom (called a pedunculated fibroid). The medical term for it is a leiomyoma or myoma.

Gestational trophoblast neoplasia (GTN): A very rare group of tumors that can grow from cells inside a woman's uterus.

Grade: A term used to describe what cancer cells look like under the microscope and the degree to which they appear abnormal.

Gynecologic oncologists: Surgeons who can perform this type of "staging" surgery for patients with endometrial cancer.

Hematogenous dissemination: Process in which cancer spreads by passing through the blood supply.

Hereditary non-polyposis colorectal cancer syndrome (HNPCC): An inherited syndrome that will increase your risk of uterine cancer.

Hospice: Also called end-of-life care, including medical, social, and religious aspects of life.

Hydatidiform mole: The result that most often develops when either one or two sperm cells fertilize an "empty" egg cell (a cell that contains no nucleus or DNA).

Hysteroscopy: A tool used to help direct the curettage in which a fiber-optic scope is used to look inside the uterus.

Ileoconduit: A small urine reservoir that is surgically created from a segment of bowel.

Ileostomy: A surgical opening constructed by bringing the end or loop of small intestine (the ileum) out onto the surface of the skin.

Intensity modulated radiation therapy (IMRT): A form of external radiation that allows for precise planning of radiation treatment, with an aim to spare normal tissue as much as possible.

Intubation: A tube inserted into a patient's throat to help her breathe.

Invasion: Growth of cancer cells into the underlying normal tissue.

Laparotomy: An incision in the abdomen, through which the uterus is removed.

Leiomyoma: Benign tumor of smooth muscle, usually the uterus. Also referred to as myoma.

Leiomyosarcoma: A type of muscular cancer of the uterus, which can sometimes present as a previously diagnosed fibroid that appears to grow far too quickly.

Lymph nodes: Bean sized organs that are part of the immune system and present throughout the body.

Lymphatic system: The "cleaning system" of the body.

Lymphedema: Swelling in the feet or legs that a woman may experience after a lymph node dissection.

Lymphocyst: A collection of fluid-filled pockets in the area of a lymph node removal.

Lymphoma: Primary lymph cancer.

Magnetic resonance imaging (MRI): MRI uses radio waves traveling through a magnetic field to significantly make out what is being imaged (that is, what is normal versus abnormal and how they relate to each other).

Malignant: Cancerous. A growth with a tendency to invade and destroy nearby tissue and spread to other parts of the body.

Maximal tolerated dose: In clinical trials, the dose level where serious side effects emerge.

Mediport: A temporary device that is surgically implanted in the chest or arm to accept an IV during chemotherapy.

Metastasis: The spreading of a disease (especially cancer) to another part of the body.

Microsatellite instability (MSI): Predisposition to certain cancers that runs in some families caused by passage of a DNA mutation.

Molar pregnancy: Pregnancy that results from abnormal development of the trophoblast.

Mutation: Changes in cell DNA which can allow irregular cell growth and division.

Myometrium: The muscular layer of the uterus that lies behind the endometrium.

Nidus: A central point or locus of an infection.

Omentum: The fatty apron surrounding the bowels.

Oophorectomy: Surgical removal of one or both ovaries.

Palliative care: The active management of patients at the end of life in which death is not viewed as something to be avoided, but is embraced as a part of the normal cycle of life.

Pap smear or **Pap test:** A procedure done during a pelvic examination at both gynecology and primary care physicians' offices. It involves a speculum exam which is how your doctor can see the cervix.

Percutaneous endoscopic gastrostomy (PEG): A tube placed by a gastrointestinal (GI) specialist in an outpatient procedure. In the context of a chronic bowel obstruction, the purpose of a PEG tube is to provide an alternative way for fluid to go, instead of vomiting to provide relief for the woman who has a chronic bowel obstruction.

Pipelle biopsy: Biopsy performed in the physician's office with a soft plastic straw called a pipelle.

Placental site trophoblastic tumor (PSTT): A tumor that develops from the place where the placenta attaches to the endometrium.

Platinum salts: Drugs that commonly serve as the basis for treatment of endometrial cancer.

Preimplantation genetic analysis: The study of fertilized eggs (or embryos) to identify normal versus abnormal embryos.

Pro-drug: A drug which is converted by the patient's liver into an anti-cancer drug after it enters the body.

Radiation: Treatment that is given to a particular part of the body in order to kill cancer cells.

Radiotherapy: Treatment of disease (especially cancer) by exposure to a radioactive substance.

Sarcoma: Tumor that develops out of the muscle or supporting tissue of the uterus.

Stage of cancer: Refers to how much of the body is involved at the time of diagnosis.

Stroma: Supporting tissue of the uterus.

Surgical menopause: When both ovaries are removed so hormones are no longer produced.

Third spacing: Fluid shift into the soft tissue, sometimes caused by TPN.

Thromboembolic events: Blood clots.

Total parenteral nutrition (TPN): A method used to provide the patient whose bowels no longer work with nutrition at the end of life, so that she does not starve to death.

Trophoblast: Specialized cells that normally surround an embryo and ultimately make the placenta that will feed the fetus during the pregnancy.

Type I endometrial cancer: Caused by an excess of the hormone estrogen.

Type II cancers: These are not associated with excess estrogen, and are usually more aggressive.

World Health Organization (WHO) scoring system: System used to assist in choosing appropriate treatment for women with persistent or metastatic disease.

INDEX

Index

Index

Other books in the *100 Questions & Answers* series

CPSIA information can be obtained
at www.ICGtesting.com
Printed in the USA
FSOW04n2028281116
27933FS